METABOLIC CONFUSION DIET

FOOD LIST FOR ENDOMORPH

The Comprehensive List of Foods to Eat and Avoid to Beat the Body at it's own Game

HILDA M. JACOBS

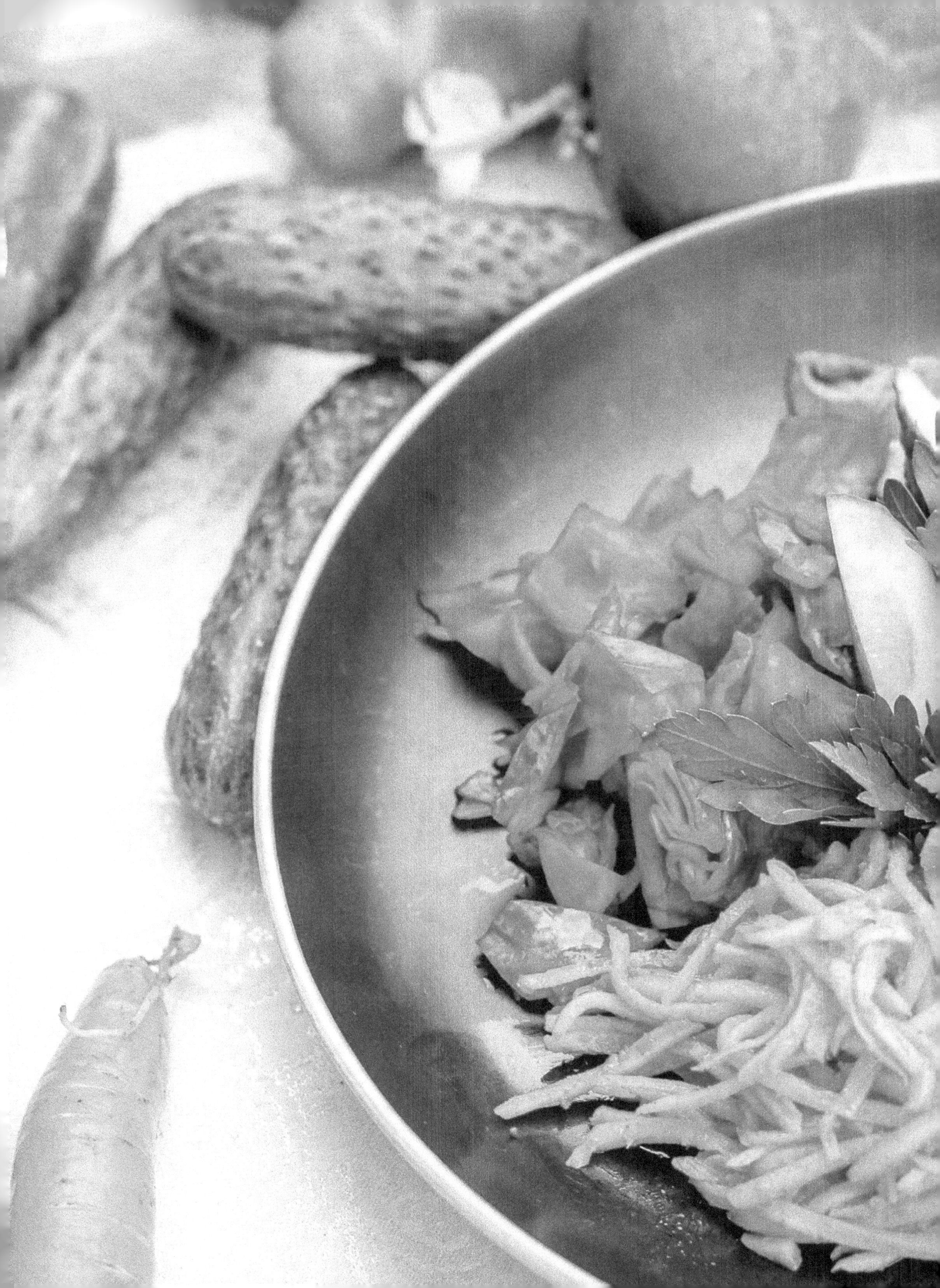

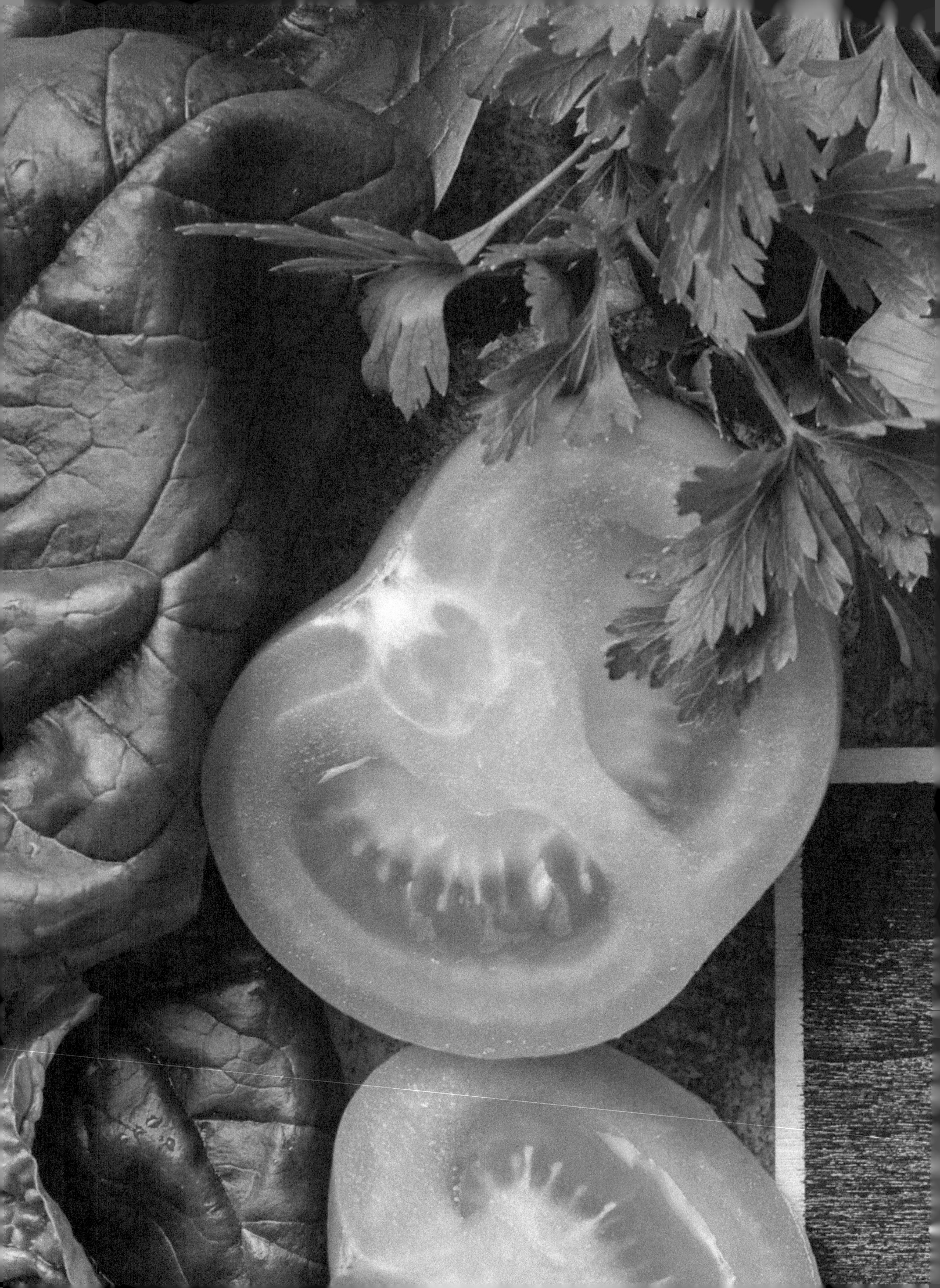

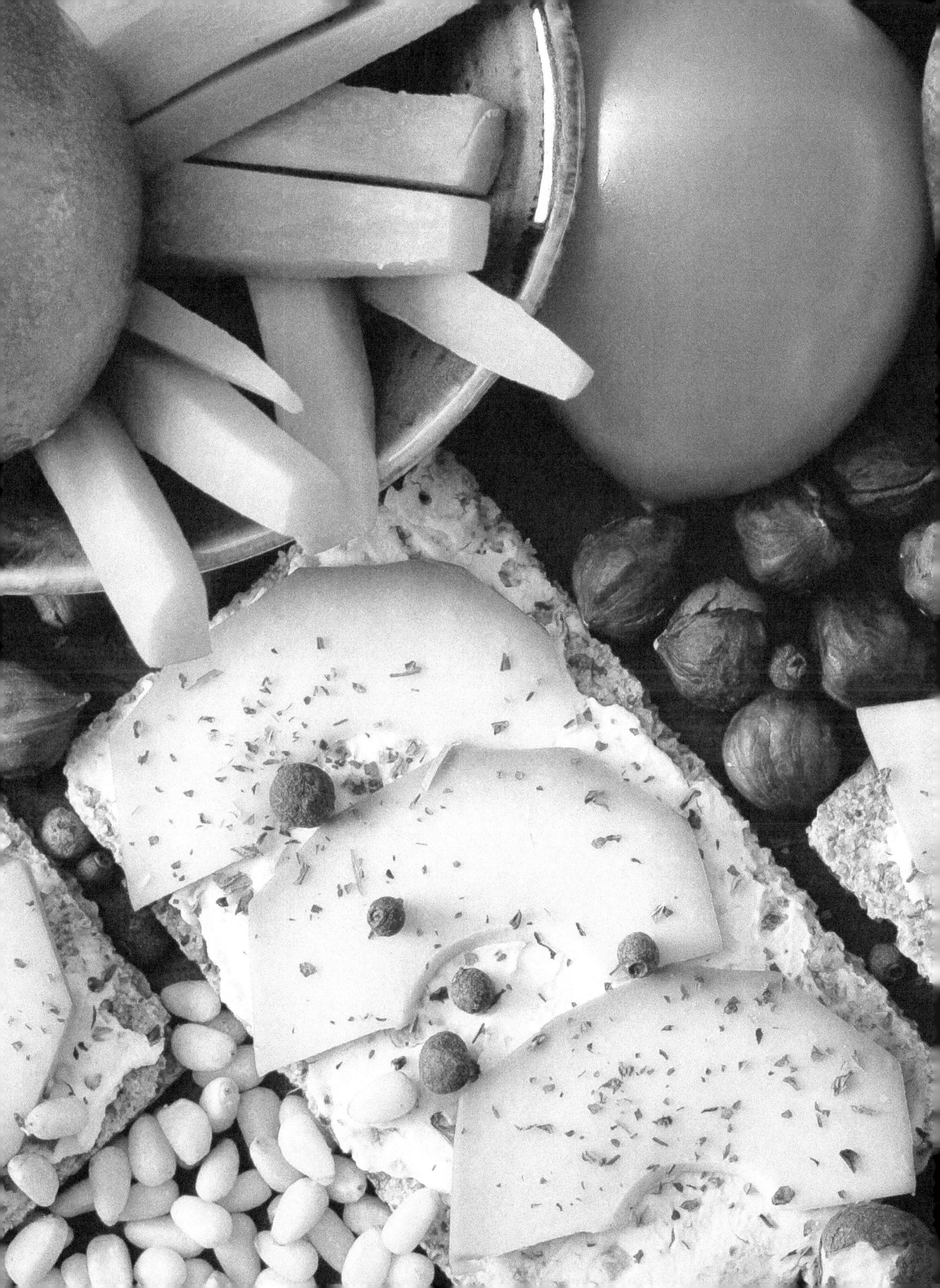

CONTENTS

INTRODUCTION

Embarking on a journey toward better health and fitness can often feel like navigating through a labyrinth of conflicting advice and fleeting trends. Among the myriad of dietary approaches that promise transformative results, the Metabolic Confusion Diet has emerged as a beacon of hope for many, especially for those identifying with the endomorph body type. In this book, "Metabolic Confusion Diet Food List for Endomorphs," we delve into a meticulously curated guide designed not only to illuminate the path toward optimal health for endomorphs but also to revolutionize the way we understand and engage with food and our metabolism.

The concept of metabolic confusion, at its core, is about outsmarting our body's natural tendencies to adapt to dietary patterns. It's a strategic deviation from the monotonous calorie-counting and restrictive eating habits that have long dominated the dieting landscape. Instead of steering you toward a one-size-fits-all regimen, we embrace the uniqueness of your metabolic blueprint—acknowledging that the endomorph body type has its specific needs and responses to food.

For those who might feel a sense of camaraderie with the term 'endomorph,' understanding your body's predisposition to storing fat over muscle can be both a revelation and a relief. It's a recognition of the fact that your journey to health is yours alone, distinct from the ectomorphs and mesomorphs of the world. This realization is not a sentence but a starting point for personalized nutrition that speaks to your body's language. Our aim is to equip you with the knowledge and tools to navigate this journey with confidence, transforming challenges into stepping stones toward your wellness goals.

"Metabolic Confusion Diet Food List for Endomorphs" is more than just a compilation of foods; it's a compass that guides you through the principles of metabolic confusion, tailored specifically for the endomorph body type. We dive into the scientific underpinnings that make metabolic confusion a viable strategy for overcoming weight loss plateaus, enhancing metabolic flexibility, and fostering a healthier relationship with food. By alternating between periods of higher and lower calorie intake, we encourage your metabolism to remain in a state of gentle flux, optimizing fat loss and muscle gain without the stagnation often encountered in traditional diets.

This book is crafted with the understanding that the journey toward health is as much about the mental and emotional aspects as it is about the physical. We recognize the frustration that can stem from following diet after diet, only to find yourself back at square one, feeling defeated and disillusioned. It's a cycle that many have endured, and it's precisely this cycle that we aim to break. By introducing variety, flexibility, and personalization into your diet, we aspire to rekindle your enthusiasm for nourishment, making eating a joyous and life-affirming act rather than a source of stress.

Within these pages, you will find a comprehensive list of foods, thoughtfully selected to resonate with the metabolic needs and preferences of endomorphs. But it's not merely about what you eat; it's also about when and how. We explore the importance of macronutrient balance, nutrient timing, and portion control, offering practical strategies that can be seamlessly integrated into your daily life. Each suggestion is rooted in the understanding that life is dynamic, and flexibility is key to sustainable success.

Our goal is to foster a sense of empowerment, enabling you to make informed decisions about your diet that align with your body type, lifestyle, and personal preferences. "Metabolic Confusion Diet Food List for Endomorphs" is designed to be a living document, one that you can return to time and again, finding new insights and inspirations as you progress along your path to wellness. It's a testament to the belief that with the right knowledge and tools, anyone can unlock their body's potential for vibrant health.

We approach the topic of metabolic confusion and endomorph nutrition with a blend of scientific rigor and empathetic understanding. It's a dialogue between us, rooted in the latest research and clinical insights, yet communicated with the warmth and clarity of a trusted friend. We're here to demystify the complexities of metabolism and dieting, presenting information in a way that's accessible, relatable, and, above all, actionable.

UNDERSTANDING METABOLIC CONFUSION

The Metabolic Confusion Diet Explained

In the realm of nutritional science, the metabolic confusion diet emerges as a novel approach designed to outsmart the body's metabolic processes. This diet, often enveloped in intrigue, is predicated on the concept of varying caloric intake to prevent the metabolism from settling into a predictable pattern. Unlike traditional diets that endorse a consistent caloric deficit or surplus, metabolic confusion alternates between periods of higher and lower calorie consumption. This method is believed to enhance metabolic flexibility, thereby facilitating more efficient fat loss and muscle gain.

At its core, the metabolic confusion diet is not merely about oscillating caloric intake; it is a strategic manipulation of the body's energy-processing systems. By varying the amount of energy supplied to the body, it purportedly keeps the metabolic rate from plateauing, a common issue in prolonged dieting scenarios. The rationale is straightforward: when the body becomes accustomed to a certain level of caloric intake, it adjusts its metabolic rate to match this intake, potentially slowing down weight loss and making dietary efforts less effective over time.

Implementing the metabolic confusion diet requires a nuanced understanding of one's own body and its caloric needs. Individuals start by determining their maintenance calorie level—the number of calories required to maintain their current weight. From this baseline, they alternate between periods of eating more calories (often termed 'high-calorie days') and eating fewer calories ('low-calorie days'). This fluctuation can be planned on a weekly or monthly basis, depending on personal preferences and goals.

The high-calorie days are not an open invitation to indulge in unhealthy foods but rather an opportunity to fuel the body with nutrient-dense calories that support muscle growth and recovery. Conversely, low-calorie days are designed to promote fat loss by creating a caloric deficit, encouraging the body to use stored fat as an energy source. This dynamic approach to calorie intake is aimed at optimizing body composition—increasing muscle mass while decreasing fat mass.

Adopting the metabolic confusion diet also involves a balanced intake of macronutrients—proteins, carbohydrates, and fats—regardless of the calorie count for the day. This balance ensures that the body receives all the necessary nutrients to function optimally, further supporting metabolic health. Protein, in particular, is emphasized for its role in muscle repair and growth, especially on high-calorie days.

This dietary strategy represents a departure from the monotonous caloric restriction models, introducing a flexible and adaptive approach to weight management. By keeping the metabolism guessing, the metabolic confusion diet aims to circumvent the adaptive responses that often lead to weight loss plateaus, making it an intriguing option for those who have found little success with traditional diets.

Differentiating Metabolic Confusion from Other Dietary Approaches

Static vs. Dynamic Caloric Intake

Traditional diets often rely on a static caloric intake model, prescribing a fixed calorie count per day aimed at creating a consistent caloric deficit for weight loss or a surplus for muscle gain. This approach, while effective for some, does not account for the body's adaptive metabolic responses over time. In contrast, the metabolic confusion diet adopts a dynamic caloric intake strategy, fluctuating between higher and lower calorie days. This variability is designed to prevent metabolic adaptation, potentially leading to more sustainable weight management and body composition improvements.

The Metabolic Confusion Diet vs. Intermittent Fasting

Intermittent fasting focuses on the timing of meals, cycling between periods of eating and fasting. While it alters when you eat, it does not inherently dictate variations in daily caloric intake or nutritional composition. The metabolic confusion diet, however, specifically targets the amount of energy consumed, irrespective of the eating window. Both strategies aim to enhance metabolic efficiency but from different angles: intermittent fasting through meal timing and metabolic confusion through caloric variability.

The Metabolic Confusion Diet vs. Carb Cycling

Carb cycling is another dietary strategy that involves alternating between high and low carbohydrate intake days, primarily to maximize fat loss and muscle gain. While carb cycling shares the principle of dietary fluctuation with metabolic confusion, it specifically manipulates carbohydrate intake rather than overall calories. The metabolic confusion diet encompasses a broader spectrum of nutritional variability, not just carbs, allowing for a more comprehensive approach to metabolic adaptation.

The Role of Personalization

A significant advantage of the metabolic confusion diet is its capacity for personalization. Unlike one-size-fits-all dietary plans, metabolic confusion allows for adjustments based on individual metabolic rates, lifestyle, activity levels, and personal goals. This personalized approach not only enhances the diet's effectiveness but also increases adherence by accommodating personal preferences and nutritional needs.

Evidence-Based Practice

While numerous diets claim to be grounded in science, the metabolic confusion diet is distinct in its approach to leveraging the body's natural metabolic processes. By understanding and applying the principles of metabolic adaptation, this diet seeks to optimize the body's energy utilization for improved health outcomes. This scientific underpinning sets it apart from diets based more on anecdotal success than on understanding human physiology.

In comparing the metabolic confusion diet to other dietary approaches, it's clear that its unique strategy of caloric fluctuation offers a novel method for addressing the challenges of weight management and metabolic health. By embracing the body's natural metabolic rhythms and manipulating them to one's advantage, the metabolic confusion diet presents a promising alternative for those seeking a flexible and effective dietary strategy.

The Science behind Metabolic Confusion: Principles and Evidence

At the heart of metabolic confusion is the principle of metabolic adaptation. The human body is remarkably adept at adjusting its metabolic rate based on caloric intake and expenditure. When calories are scarce, the body can slow down its metabolic processes to conserve energy, a survival mechanism rooted in our evolutionary history. Conversely, when calorie intake is abundant, the metabolism can increase to handle the excess energy. Metabolic confusion leverages this adaptability by systematically varying caloric intake, aiming to keep the metabolism in a state of flux to prevent the slowdown associated with prolonged calorie restriction.

Metabolic flexibility refers to the body's ability to efficiently switch between fuel sources (such as carbohydrates and fats) based on availability and demand. An optimized metabolic flexibility is associated with improved energy levels, better weight management, and a reduced risk of metabolic diseases. The metabolic confusion diet, with its cyclical approach to calorie consumption, is theorized to enhance this flexibility, enabling the body to more adeptly handle dietary variations and utilize different energy sources.

While direct studies on metabolic confusion are still emerging, related research provides supportive insights. Studies on intermittent fasting and varying meal patterns have shown potential benefits for metabolism and weight management, suggesting that disrupting the body's metabolic expectations can have positive effects. Additionally, research on the benefits of periodic refeeding (increasing caloric intake after a period of restriction) indicates that strategic increases in calories can temporarily boost metabolic rate and improve leptin sensitivity, a hormone critical to hunger regulation and metabolic rate.

Evidence from individuals and practitioners who have implemented the metabolic confusion diet points to several potential benefits, including improved weight loss outcomes, better maintenance of muscle mass during dieting, and increased dietary adherence due to the flexibility of the approach. While individual results can vary, the principle of introducing variability into one's diet appears to mitigate some of the common pitfalls associated with traditional dieting, such as metabolic slowdown, weight loss plateaus, and diminished motivation.

It's important to acknowledge that while the foundational principles of metabolic confusion are supported by existing metabolic and nutritional science, comprehensive research specifically targeting the metabolic confusion diet is needed. Future studies should aim to quantify the effects of metabolic confusion on weight loss, body composition, metabolic health markers, and long-term adherence to better understand its place in nutritional science and practice.

Tailoring Nutrition to Body Type

The nutritional approach for endomorphs emphasizes managing calorie intake, focusing on macronutrient distribution, and choosing foods that support metabolic health. Here's how to structure your diet for optimal results:

1. Managing Caloric Intake

For endomorphs, finding the right caloric balance is crucial. Consuming fewer calories than expended is necessary for weight loss, but it's important to avoid drastic reductions that could slow metabolism further. A moderate deficit, tailored to individual activity levels and metabolic rates, promotes sustainable weight loss.

2. Macronutrient Distribution

Protein: High protein intake is essential for endomorphs. Protein supports muscle maintenance and growth, increases satiety, and has a higher thermic effect, meaning it burns more calories during digestion. Aim for lean sources like poultry, fish, legumes, and low-fat dairy.

Carbohydrates: Carbs should be consumed mindfully, focusing on low-glycemic options that provide sustained energy and minimize insulin spikes. Whole grains, vegetables, and fruits rich in fiber are ideal choices.

Fats: Healthy fats are vital for hormone regulation and satiety. Incorporate sources like avocados, nuts, seeds, and olive oil, keeping an eye on portion sizes due to their high-calorie content.

3. Emphasizing Nutrient-Dense Foods

Endomorphs benefit from a diet rich in nutrient-dense foods. These foods provide essential vitamins, minerals, and antioxidants without excessive calories, supporting overall health and aiding in weight management.

4. Timing and Frequency of Meals

Meal timing can influence metabolic rate and hunger levels. Eating smaller, balanced meals every 3-4 hours can help maintain steady energy levels and prevent overeating. Including a protein source at each meal is beneficial for muscle maintenance and satiety.

Deciphering Body Composition: Tools and Techniques

1. Bioelectrical Impedance Analysis (BIA)

Bioelectrical Impedance Analysis is a widely accessible and non-invasive method for estimating body composition. By sending a weak electrical current through the body and measuring the resistance (impedance) encountered by the current, BIA estimates the volume of fat mass and lean mass. Since the electrical current travels faster through muscle (which contains more water) than fat, this method can provide a quick estimate of body fat percentage. Advanced BIA devices can also segment the body into parts (arms, legs, and trunk), offering more detailed insights.

Despite its convenience, the accuracy of BIA can be affected by hydration levels, meal consumption, and skin temperature. Therefore, it's recommended to follow standardized testing conditions for consistent results.

2. Dual-Energy X-ray Absorptiometry (DEXA)

Originally developed to assess bone density, DEXA has become a gold standard for comprehensive body composition analysis. By using low-dose x-rays at two different energy levels, DEXA scans can differentiate between bone mass, lean mass, and fat mass throughout the entire body. It provides detailed images that allow for the analysis of regional body composition, making it invaluable for understanding fat distribution patterns and assessing skeletal health.

The precision and detail of DEXA scans come with a higher cost and the need for specialized equipment, usually found in medical facilities or research institutions. Despite this, its accuracy and reliability make it a preferred choice for those seeking detailed assessments.

3. Skin Calipers

Skinfold measurements with calipers are one of the oldest and most straightforward techniques for estimating body fat percentage. By measuring the thickness of skinfolds at specific sites on the body, practitioners can estimate overall body fat. This method relies on the assumption that a certain proportion of the total body fat is subcutaneous and can be captured by skinfold measurements.

Although caliper measurements can vary based on the skill of the practitioner and the quality of the calipers, this method is cost-effective and widely used, especially in field settings. When performed consistently by a trained professional, skin calipers can provide a reliable estimate of body fat changes over time.

4. Hydrostatic Weighing

Often referred to as underwater weighing, hydrostatic weighing was once considered the gold standard for measuring body composition. This technique measures a person's body density by determining body volume through displacement after submerging in water. Given the different densities of fat mass and lean mass, this method can accurately estimate body fat percentage.

While hydrostatic weighing provides high accuracy, it requires specialized equipment, trained personnel, and the willingness of the individual to be submerged in water. These factors limit its accessibility and convenience for routine use.

5. Air Displacement Plethysmography (ADP)

ADP, best known by the brand name Bod Pod, uses air displacement to determine body volume and, subsequently, body density. By sitting inside a small chamber, the volume of air displaced by the person is measured, which is then used to calculate body density and, by extension, body composition.

This method offers several advantages, including ease of use, non-invasiveness, and quick measurement time. It's particularly useful for populations where other methods might be challenging to implement, such as in obese individuals or those with mobility issues.

6. 3D Body Scanners

Emerging technology in the form of 3D body scanners offers a novel approach to assessing body composition and shape. By capturing a three-dimensional image of the body, these scanners can measure circumferences, volume, and surface area with high precision. While not directly measuring body fat or muscle mass, the data obtained can be used to estimate body composition and changes over time, providing valuable feedback for fitness and health interventions.

7. Magnetic Resonance Imaging (MRI) and Computed Tomography (CT)

MRI and CT scans provide the most detailed images of body composition, allowing for the visualization of internal structures, including muscle tissue, fat deposits, and even organ fat. These techniques are invaluable for research and clinical assessments of body composition, particularly in understanding the distribution of visceral fat, which is linked to various metabolic diseases.

However, the high cost, need for specialized equipment, and exposure to radiation (in the case of CT scans) limit their use to specific clinical or research applications rather than routine body composition assessments.

Metabolism Uncovered: Mechanisms and Influences

The Basic Mechanisms of Metabolism

Metabolism can be broken down into two fundamental processes: catabolism and anabolism. Catabolism involves the breakdown of molecules to extract energy, whereas anabolism uses this energy to synthesize all compounds needed by the cells.

1. **Catabolism**: This process is akin to a controlled demolition, breaking down complex molecules like carbohydrates, fats, and proteins into simpler ones such as glucose, fatty acids, and amino acids, respectively. The pinnacle of catabolism is cellular respiration, a process that converts glucose into adenosine triphosphate (ATP), the energy currency of the cell.

2. **Anabolism**: Contrasting catabolism, anabolism is the construction crew of metabolism, using energy to build complex molecules from simpler ones. These processes are crucial for cell growth, repair, and reproduction, synthesizing essential components like proteins, nucleic acids, and lipids.

The Role of Enzymes in Metabolism

Enzymes are the unsung heroes of metabolism, acting as catalysts that significantly speed up the rate of biochemical reactions. Each enzyme is specific to a particular reaction, ensuring that metabolic processes occur swiftly and efficiently. The regulation of these enzymes, and hence metabolic pathways, is tightly controlled by the body to meet its immediate needs, illustrating the remarkable adaptability of our metabolic systems.

Influences on Metabolism

Several factors influence the efficiency and direction of metabolic processes, including but not limited to genetics, age, sex, hormone levels, and lifestyle factors like diet and exercise.

1. **Genetics**: Our genetic makeup plays a foundational role in determining our metabolic rate and how we metabolize different nutrients. Genetic variations can affect how quickly or slowly we process foods, influencing body weight, energy levels, and risk of metabolic diseases.

2. **Age**: As we age, our metabolism naturally slows down, partly due to a decrease in muscle mass and changes in hormone levels. This decline makes it increasingly important to stay active and adjust dietary habits to maintain a healthy metabolic rate.

3. **Sex**: Generally, men have a faster metabolism than women, largely because they have more muscle mass, which burns more calories at rest. Hormonal differences also contribute to variations in metabolic rate between sexes.

4. **Hormones**: Hormones like thyroid hormones, insulin, and cortisol play critical roles in regulating metabolism. For example, thyroid hormones regulate metabolic rate, insulin controls blood sugar levels, and cortisol, the stress hormone, can influence energy storage and expenditure.

5. **Diet**: What we eat can directly impact our metabolism. Diets rich in protein can increase the thermic effect of food, slightly boosting metabolic rate. Conversely, overconsumption of sugary and highly processed foods can disrupt insulin sensitivity, leading to metabolic issues.

6. **Physical Activity**: Regular exercise is a potent stimulator of metabolism. Not only does physical activity burn calories, but it also builds muscle mass, which in turn increases resting metabolic rate, allowing the body to burn more calories even at rest.

Adapting to Maximize Metabolic Health

Understanding the intricacies of metabolism and the factors influencing it empowers us to make informed decisions about our health. Here are a few strategies to support and optimize metabolic health:

- **Balanced Nutrition**: Emphasize a diet rich in whole foods, with a good balance of macronutrients (carbohydrates, proteins, and fats) and essential micronutrients (vitamins and minerals) to support metabolic processes.

- **Regular Exercise**: Incorporate both resistance training to build muscle and cardiovascular exercises to improve heart health and stamina, boosting your metabolic rate.

- **Adequate Sleep**: Ensure sufficient sleep each night, as sleep deprivation can disrupt metabolic health, affecting hormone levels and increasing the risk of obesity and diabetes.

- **Stress Management**: Chronic stress can negatively impact metabolic health through the overproduction of cortisol. Techniques such as mindfulness, meditation, and regular physical activity can help manage stress levels.

- **Hydration**: Drinking enough water is essential for optimal metabolic function. Hydration aids in energy production and helps the body process nutrients more efficiently.

Customizing Your Diet: Strategies for Personalization

The foundation of any personalized diet begins with understanding your body's specific nutritional needs. These needs are influenced by a myriad of factors including age, gender, weight, height, physical activity level, and health goals, whether they be weight loss, muscle gain, maintenance, or improving overall health markers. Utilizing tools such as the Harris-Benedict equation can provide a baseline for caloric needs, which is then adjusted based on activity levels and goals. However, calories only tell part of the story; the quality of calories consumed is equally crucial. This means focusing on nutrient-dense foods that provide vitamins, minerals, antioxidants, and other nutrients essential for optimal health.

Genetic Influences and Bioindividuality

Emerging research in nutrigenomics has begun to shed light on how our genes can affect our nutritional needs and how we respond to different foods. For example, variations in the MTHFR gene can affect how the body processes folate, while the APOE gene can influence fat metabolism, impacting cardiovascular health. Understanding these genetic nuances can guide more personalized nutrition planning, emphasizing or limiting certain nutrients to cater to one's genetic profile.

Metabolic Typing and Hormonal Considerations

Metabolic typing is a concept that suggests individuals metabolize macronutrients differently, which can influence optimal dietary composition. While research in this area is ongoing, it offers a lens through which to view the customization of diet—some may thrive on a higher carbohydrate diet, while others may require higher levels of protein or fat to feel their best. Similarly, hormonal imbalances, such as insulin resistance or thyroid disorders, necessitate adjustments in dietary composition to manage and mitigate health impacts effectively.

The Role of Gut Health

The microbiome is a complex ecosystem within the gut, playing a pivotal role in health and disease. The composition of gut flora can influence digestion, immunity, and even mental health. Customizing your diet to support gut health involves incorporating a variety of fiber-rich foods, fermented foods, and potentially, targeted probiotics. This not only aids in digestion but can also have far-reaching effects on overall health.

Tailoring Your Diet: Practical Steps

1. **Self-Monitoring and Journaling**: Begin by tracking your food intake, noting not only what you eat but how you feel afterward. This can help identify foods that energize, satisfy, or perhaps lead to discomfort or energy slumps.

2. **Experimentation and Adjustment**: Based on your observations, start experimenting by adjusting macronutrient ratios, incorporating new foods, and observing changes in your body and energy levels. It's a process of trial and error, guided by personal feedback.

3. **Seek Professional Guidance**: Consider consulting with a dietitian or nutritionist who can provide insights into your nutritional needs and help tailor your diet based on detailed assessments, including possibly genetic testing and metabolic rate measurements.

4. **Incorporating Variety**: Ensure your diet includes a wide range of foods to not only prevent boredom but also to provide a broad spectrum of nutrients. This involves experimenting with different vegetables, fruits, proteins, whole grains, and healthy fats.

5. **Monitoring and Reevaluation**: Your body changes over time, and so do your nutritional needs. Regularly assess your diet's effectiveness in meeting your health goals and make adjustments as needed. This includes revisiting your caloric needs, macronutrient distribution, and the inclusion of specific foods that support your health objectives.

CORE PRINCIPLES OF ENDOMORPH NUTRITION

Understanding the Roles of Macronutrients

1. **Carbohydrates**: Often misrepresented as the enemy of weight loss, carbohydrates are actually the body's primary energy source. They fuel brain activity, support bodily functions, and enhance physical performance. The key lies in selecting high-quality, fiber-rich carbohydrates such as whole grains, vegetables, fruits, and legumes, which provide sustained energy and support metabolic health.

2. **Proteins**: Essential for the repair and growth of tissues, proteins also play a crucial role in weight management. They provide the building blocks for muscles, support immune function, and contribute to a feeling of satiety. High-protein diets have been linked to increased metabolic rate and reduced appetite, making protein a critical component of a weight management strategy.

3. **Fats**: Long vilified in the diet culture, fats are essential for numerous bodily functions, including hormone production, nutrient absorption, and cell structure. Healthy fats, particularly those from plant sources and fatty fish, support heart health, enhance satiety, and can prevent overeating. The focus should be on monounsaturated and polyunsaturated fats, while minimizing trans fats and saturated fats from processed foods.

Customizing Your Macronutrient Ratio

The ideal macronutrient ratio can vary significantly among individuals, influenced by factors such as age, gender, activity level, and personal health goals. However, a starting point for those looking to optimize health and weight might be:

- **Carbohydrates**: 45-65% of total daily calories
- **Proteins**: 20-35% of total daily calories
- **Fats**: 20-35% of total daily calories

This distribution can serve as a guideline, but it's crucial to adjust based on personal preferences, metabolic responses, and nutritional needs.

Strategies for Balancing Macronutrients

1. **Listen to Your Body**: Monitoring how your body responds to different macronutrient distributions can provide invaluable insights. Some may thrive on a higher carbohydrate intake, while others may find a lower carbohydrate, higher fat and protein diet more beneficial for satiety and weight management.

2. **Consider Your Activity Level**: Those engaged in high levels of physical activity, particularly endurance sports, may require a higher intake of carbohydrates to support energy needs. Conversely,

individuals with a more sedentary lifestyle might benefit from a lower carbohydrate intake, prioritizing protein and healthy fats to manage weight and metabolic health.

3. **Quality over Quantity**: Focusing on the quality of macronutrients can significantly impact health outcomes. Opt for whole, unprocessed foods to maximize nutrient density and minimize added sugars and refined carbohydrates, which can contribute to weight gain and metabolic issues.

4. **Timing Matters**: Nutrient timing can also influence metabolic outcomes. Consuming protein-rich foods after a workout can aid muscle recovery, while incorporating a balanced meal with carbohydrates, protein, and fats can sustain energy levels throughout the day.

Macronutrients and Weight Management

Balancing macronutrients is not just about weight loss but about optimizing body composition—increasing muscle mass while reducing fat mass. This approach supports metabolic health, enhances physical performance, and improves overall well-being.

1. **High-Protein Diets**: Research consistently shows that higher protein intakes can support weight loss efforts by enhancing satiety, reducing appetite, and increasing the thermic effect of food (the energy required to digest, absorb, and metabolize nutrients).

2. **Low-Glycemic Carbohydrates**: Choosing carbohydrates with a low glycemic index can help manage blood sugar levels, reduce hunger, and support sustained energy, aiding in weight management and reducing the risk of metabolic diseases.

3. **Healthy Fats**: Incorporating healthy fats into the diet can also support weight management efforts. Fats are more energy-dense but also highly satiating, which can help prevent overeating and snack cravings.

The Role of Nutrient Timing in Metabolic Regulation

At the heart of nutrient timing is the synchronization of nutrient intake with the body's natural rhythms and activities. This strategy leverages the anabolic (building) and catabolic (breaking down) phases of metabolism, aiming to enhance muscle synthesis, energy utilization, and recovery, while minimizing fat storage. The foundational principles of nutrient timing revolve around three critical windows: the pre-workout or energy phase, the post-workout or anabolic phase, and the recovery phase.

1. **Pre-Workout (Energy Phase)**: The primary objective during this phase is to fuel the body for optimal performance. Consuming a balanced meal of carbohydrates and proteins 2-3 hours before exercise can provide sustained energy and prevent muscle catabolism. For those who train early or can't consume a full meal, a small snack rich in easily digestible carbohydrates 30 minutes prior can suffice.

2. **Post-Workout (Anabolic Phase)**: The 30 to 60 minutes following exercise, often referred to as the "anabolic window," is crucial for recovery and muscle growth. During this window, the body's ability

to replenish glycogen stores and absorb amino acids is enhanced. A post-workout meal or snack high in carbohydrates and protein can expedite recovery, support muscle repair, and reduce soreness.

3. **Recovery Phase**: This phase focuses on the broader period of recovery that extends beyond the immediate post-workout window. Here, the emphasis is on balanced meals that support muscle repair, replenish glycogen stores, and ensure overall recovery. Quality sleep and hydration are also integral components of the recovery phase, as they significantly impact metabolic health and performance.

Nutrient Timing and Metabolic Regulation

The strategic timing of nutrient intake can significantly influence metabolic regulation, impacting everything from glycemic control to fat metabolism. For individuals with metabolic concerns such as insulin resistance, timed nutrient intake can help stabilize blood glucose levels, reducing spikes and crashes that can lead to increased fat storage and cravings.

Moreover, nutrient timing can optimize the body's use of fats and carbohydrates as energy sources. By aligning carbohydrate intake with periods of high activity, the body is more likely to use glucose efficiently, minimizing the likelihood of fat storage. Conversely, increasing the intake of healthy fats and proteins during less active periods can support sustained energy levels and satiety, preventing overeating and promoting a healthier body composition.

Practical Applications of Nutrient Timing

Implementing nutrient timing into one's dietary strategy requires consideration of individual goals, lifestyles, and metabolic health. For those aiming to improve body composition, focusing on the post-workout anabolic window to maximize muscle recovery and growth can be particularly beneficial. Individuals looking to enhance endurance and performance may prioritize the pre-workout energy phase to ensure adequate fueling for sustained activity.

It's also essential to consider the quality of nutrients consumed. High-glycemic carbohydrates may be suitable for immediate post-workout recovery, but complex carbohydrates, lean proteins, and healthy fats should constitute the bulk of one's diet to support overall metabolic health and wellness.

Mastering Portion Control: Techniques and Importance

The Significance of Portion Control

Understanding the importance of portion control is the first step toward nutritional empowerment. In a world where food portions have steadily increased, especially in restaurant settings, our perception of what constitutes a "normal" serving size has become distorted. This escalation in portion sizes has paralleled rising rates of obesity and related health issues, highlighting the need for a recalibration of our eating habits.

Portion control is instrumental in regulating energy intake, which is crucial for weight management and the prevention of chronic diseases such as diabetes, heart disease, and certain cancers. By mastering portion control, individuals can ensure they consume enough nutrients to support their body's needs without excess caloric intake that leads to weight gain and metabolic imbalances.

Techniques for Mastering Portion Control

1. **Visual Cues for Estimating Portions**: Learning to estimate serving sizes using visual cues can be a practical tool for portion control. For instance, a serving of meat should be about the size of a deck of cards, while a serving of carbohydrates, like pasta or rice, should be approximately the size of a baseball. Incorporating these visual comparisons into meal preparation can help maintain portion sizes without the need for constant measurement.

2. **Utilizing Smaller Plates and Bowls**: The psychology of eating plays a significant role in how much we consume. By using smaller plates and bowls, individuals can help control portion sizes naturally. A full smaller plate provides visual satisfaction and can lead to a reduction in caloric intake without a feeling of deprivation.

3. **Mindful Eating Practices**: Mindful eating is a technique that involves paying full attention to the experience of eating and savoring each bite. By eating slowly and without distraction, individuals are more likely to notice signals of fullness and satisfaction, reducing the likelihood of overeating.

4. **Pre-portioning Snacks**: It's easy to overeat when consuming directly from a large container or package. Pre-portioning snacks into individual servings can prevent mindless eating and help manage portion sizes effectively.

5. **Understanding and Listening to Hunger Cues**: Tuning into the body's natural hunger and satiety signals is crucial for portion control. Eating in response to hunger rather than emotional cues or out of habit encourages a more harmonious relationship with food.

6. **Strategic Leftovers**: When cooking at home or dining out, intentionally planning for leftovers can aid portion control. By setting aside a portion of the meal before beginning to eat, individuals can prevent overeating and enjoy a second meal at a later time.

FOODS TO EAT FOR ENDOMORPHS

Lean Protein

Lean Protein Source	Portion Size	Calories (kcal)	Protein (g)	Carbohydrates (g)	Fat (g)	Fiber (g)
Alligator	85g	83	25	1	1.5	1
Baked Beans (Canned)	130g	110	7	25	1.5	6
Bison	85g	94	23	1	2.5	1
Buffalo	85g	94	23	1	2.5	1
Canned Salmon (Pink)	85g	100	18	1	4.5	1
Canned Tuna (in Water)	85g	74	17	1	2	1
Chicken Thigh (Skinless)	85g	163	19	1	11	1
Chickpeas	82g	135	8	25	3.5	7
Cod	85g	90	21	1	2	1
Cottage Cheese (Low-fat)	113g	81	15	5	2	1
Edamame (Soybeans)	93g	121	12	10	6	5
Egg Whites	3 egg whites	52	12	1	1	1
Elk	85g	136	25	1	5.5	1
Flank Steak	85g	158	26	1	7	1
Greek Yogurt (Non-fat)	245g	131	24	10	1	1
Grouper	85g	101	21	1	2	1
Haddock	85g	77	19	1	1.5	1
Hake	85g	72	17	1	1.5	1
Halibut	85g	78	18	1	2	1
Kangaroo	85g	100	21	1	3	1
Lean Bison	85g	94	23	1	2.5	1

Lean Ground Beef (90% lean)	85g	181	23	1	11	1
Lean Ground Chicken	85g	138	24	1	5.5	1
Lean Ground Turkey (93% lean)	85g	136	23	1	6	1
Lean Lamb	85g	154	25	1	6.5	1
Lean Pork Chops	85g	144	24	1	6	1
Lean Veal	85g	126	25	1	4	1
Lentils	92g	116	10	21	1.5	9
Mackerel (Wild-caught)	85g	234	20	1	17	1
Mahi-Mahi	85g	86	19	1	2.5	1
Mussels	85g	74	13	5	3	1
Octopus	85g	75	16	1	2.2	1
Ostrich	85g	89	21	1	2	1
Oysters	85g	87	12	5	4	1
Pheasant	85g	135	25	1	4.5	1
Pork Loin (Center Cut)	85g	117	24	1	3	1
Pork Tenderloin	85g	123	25	1	3.5	1
Prawns	85g	85	19	1	2.5	1
Quinoa	92g	112	5	21	2.5	3.5
Rabbit	85g	174	25	1	9	1
Salmon (Wild-caught)	85g	176	19	1	12	1
Sardines (Canned in Water)	3.75 oz	88	19	1	2.5	1
Scallops	85g	76	16	4	1.5	1
Shrimp	85g	85	19	1	2.5	1
Skinless Chicken Breast	85g	129	27	1	4	1
Skinless Duck Breast	85g	136	25	1	5	1
Skinless Turkey Thigh	85g	136	27	1	3.5	1
Snapper	85g	95	21	1	2.5	1

Swordfish	85g	141	22	1	7	1
Tempeh	85g	161	16	10	10	4
Tilapia	85g	85	22	1	2.5	1
Tofu (Extra Firm)	85g	71	9	3	5	2
Trout	85g	134	21	1	6.5	1
Tuna Steak	85g	110	25	1	1.5	1
Turkey Breast	85g	136	31	1	2	1
Venison	85g	159	27	1	7	1
Yellowtail (Hamachi)	85g	111	23	1	3.5	1

Carbohydrates

Food Item	Portion Size	Calories	Carbs (g)	Fiber (g)	Protein (g)
Acorn Squash	1 cup	116	31	10	3
Alfalfa Sprouts	1 cup	9	2	2	2
Amaranth	1 cup	252	47	6	10
Apples	1 medium	96	26	5	1.5
Artichoke	1 medium	61	14	8	5
Arugula	1 cup	6	2	1	1.5
Asparagus	1 cup	28	6	4	4
Avocado	1/2 medium	121	7	6	2.5
Bamboo Shoots	1 cup	15	4	3	3
Barley	1 cup	194	46	7	4.5
Beets	1 cup	60	14	5	3
Bell Peppers	1 medium	25	7	3.1	2
Black Beans	1 cup	228	42	16	16
Black Rice	1 cup	281	65	5	7
Blackberries	1 cup	63	15	9	3
Blueberries	1 cup	85	22	4.6	2.1
Bok Choy	1 cup	10	2	2	2
Broccoli	1 cup	32	7	3.4	3.6
Brown Rice	1 cup	216	46	4.5	6
Brussels Sprouts	1 cup	39	9	4.3	4
Buckwheat	1 cup	156	34	5.5	7

Bulgur	1 cup	152	35	9	7
Butternut Squash	1 cup	83	23	8	3
Cabbage	1 cup	23	6	3	2
Cantaloupe	1 cup	55	14	2.4	2.3
Carrots	1 cup	53	13	4.6	2.2
Cassava	1 cup	331	79	5	4
Cauliflower	1 cup	26	6	3	3
Celery	1 cup	17	5	3	2
Chia Seeds	1 oz	138	13	12	5
Chickpeas	1 cup	270	46	13.5	15.5
Collard Greens	1 cup	12	3	2	2
Corn	1 medium ear	89	20	3	4
Couscous	1 cup	177	37	3	7
Cranberries	1 cup	47	13	5.6	1.4
Dragon Fruit	1 cup	61	10	2	2
Durian	1 cup	358	67	10	5
Eggplant	1 cup	21	6	3.5	1.8
Endive	1 cup	9	3	2	1.6
Escarole	1 cup	16	4	4	2
Farro	1 cup	223	40	6	9
Fennel	1 cup	28	7	4	2
Figs (Fresh)	1 medium	31	9	2	1.4
Goji Berries	1 oz	24	5	2	4
Grapefruit	1 medium	53	14	3	2
Guava	1 medium	38	9	4	2
Jackfruit	1 cup	156	41	4	4
Jerusalem Artichoke	1 cup	110	27	3	4
Jicama	1 cup	47	12	7	2
Kale	1 cup	34	7	2	4
Kiwi	1 medium	43	11	3	1.8
Leek	1 cup	55	14	3	2

Lentils	1 cup	231	41	17	19
Lotus Root	1 cup	86	21	6	3
Lychee	1 cup	126	32	3	2
Mangoes	1 cup	100	26	4	2.4
Millet	1 cup	208	42	3	7
Muesli	1/2 cup	145	31	5	5
Mulberries	1 cup	61	15	3	3
Mustard Greens	1 cup	16	3	3	3
Nectarines	1 medium	63	16	3	2
Oats	1/2 cup	155	28	5	8
Okra	1 cup	34	8	4	3
Oranges	1 medium	63	16	4	2
Papaya	1 cup	60	16	4	1.9
Parsnip	1 cup	101	25	8	2.6
Passion Fruit	1 cup	71	18	26	6
Peaches	1 medium	59	15	3	2
Pears	1 medium	103	28	7	2
Peas	1 cup	63	12	5	5
Pineapple	1 cup	83	23	3.3	1.9
Plums	1 medium	31	9	2	1.5
Pomegranate	1/2 cup	73	17	4.5	2.5
Pumpkin	1 cup	50	13	4	3
Quinoa	1 cup	223	40	6	9
Radicchio	1 cup	10	3	2	2
Radish	1 cup	20	5	3	1.8
Rambutan	1 cup	126	32	3	2
Raspberries	1 cup	65	16	9	2.5
Rutabaga	1 cup	51	12	4	2
Rye Bread	1 slice	84	16.5	2.9	3.7
Salsify	1 cup	111	27	4	4
Seaweed	1 cup	31	8	2	3

Sorghum	1 cup	652	144	13	23
Sourdough Bread	1 slice	91	19	2	5
Spelt	1 cup	247	52	8.6	11.6
Spinach	1 cup	8	2	1.7	1.9
Strawberries	1 cup	50	13	4	2
Sweet Potato	1 medium	113	27	5	3
Swiss Chard	1 cup	8	2	2	2
Taro Root	1 cup	188	46	7	2
Teff	1 cup	256	51	8	11
Turnip	1 medium	35	9	3	2
Water Chestnut	1 cup	101	25	4	3
Watercress	1 cup	5	2	1	1.8
Whole Wheat Bread	1 slice	81	16	3	5
Whole Wheat Pasta	1 cup	175	38	5	8.5
Yams	1 cup	159	38	6	3
Zucchini	1 cup	18	4	2	2.4

Fats

Food Item	Portion Size	Calories per Portion	Protein (g)	Fat (g)	Carbs (g)
Almond Butter	1 tbsp	99	3	10	4
Almonds	1 oz	161	7	15	7
Anchovies	1 oz	43	7	3	1
Avocado	1/2 medium	161	3	16	10
Avocado Oil	1 tbsp	125	1	15	1
Beef Tallow	1 tbsp	116	1	14	1
Bison	3 oz	153	23	8	1
Black Olives	10 olives	51	1	6	4
Boar	3 oz	161	25	5	1
Brazil Nuts	1 oz	188	5	20	4
Buffalo	3 oz	139	24	4	1
Cacao Nibs	1 tbsp	131	3	13	11

Camelina Oil	1 tbsp	121	1	15	1
Canola Oil	1 tbsp	125	1	15	1
Cashew Butter	1 tbsp	95	4	9	5
Cashews	1 oz	156	6	13	10
Chia Seeds	1 tbsp	59	3	5	6
Chicken Fat	1 tbsp	116	1	14	1
Clams	3 oz	127	23	3	5
Cocoa Butter	1 tbsp	121	1	15	1
Coconut Oil	1 tbsp	122	1	15	1
Cod Liver Oil	1 tsp	42	1	5.5	1
Corn Oil	1 tbsp	121	1	15	1
Cottage Cheese (Full-Fat)	1 cup	207	29	10	7
Dark Chocolate (70%+)	1 oz	171	3	13	14
Duck Breast	3 oz	133	25	4	1
Duck Fat	1 tbsp	116	1	14	1
Eel	3 oz	185	12	13	7
Eggs (whole)	1 large	73	7	6	2
Elk	3 oz	159	27	4	1
Emu	3 oz	141	25	5	1
Feta Cheese	1 oz	76	5	7	2
Flax Seeds	1 tbsp	56	3	5	4
Ghee	1 tbsp	113	1	14	1
Goat Cheese	1 oz	77	6	7	2
Grapeseed Oil	1 tbsp	121	1	15	1
Grass-fed Beef	3 oz	191	23	10	1
Greek Yogurt (Full-Fat)	1 cup	191	19	11	7
Green Olives	10 olives	43	1	5	2
Halibut	3 oz	116	23	4	1
Hazelnuts	1 oz	177	5	18	6
Hemp Seeds	1 tbsp	58	4	6	2
Herring	3 oz	174	21	11	1

Kangaroo	3 oz	99	23	2	1
Krill Oil	1 tsp	41	1	5	1
Lamb	3 oz	251	22	18	1
Lard	1 tbsp	116	1	14	1
Liver (chicken, beef)	3 oz	151	21	6	6
Macadamia Nuts	1 oz	204	3	22	5
Mackerel	3 oz	233	22	17	1
MCT Oil	1 tbsp	116	1	15	1
Mussels	85.05	147	21	5	7
Olive Oil	14.79	120	1	15	1
Oysters	85.05	88	10	4	5
Palm Oil	14.79	121	1	15	1
Peanut Butter	14.79	95	5	9	4
Peanut Oil	14.79	120	1	15	1
Pecans	28.35	197	4	21	5
Perilla Oil	14.79	121	1	15	1
Pine Nuts	28.35	192	5	20	5
Pistachios	28.35	160	7	14	9
Poppy Seeds	14.79	48	2	5	4
Poultry Skin (chicken, turkey)	28.35	116	8	11	1
Pumpkin Seeds	28.35	152	8	14	6
Quail	(varies)	138	25	4	1
Rabbit	85.05	148	29	4	1
Rice Bran Oil	14.79	121	1	15	1
Sacha Inchi Oil	14.79	121	1	15	1
Safflower Oil	14.79	121	1	15	1
Salmon	85.05	178	18	10	1
Sardines	(varies)	192	24	11	1
Sesame Oil	14.79	121	1	15	1
Sesame Seeds	14.79	53	3	6	3
Soybean Oil	14.79	121	1	15	1

Sunflower Oil	14.79	121	1	15	1
Sunflower Seeds	28.35	165	7	15	7
Tahini	14.79	90	4	9	4
Tallow	14.79	116	1	14	1
Trout	85.05	163	22	8	1
Tuna (canned, in water)	85.05	74	18	2	1
Venison	85.05	159	27	4	1
Walnut Oil	14.79	121	1	15	1
Walnuts	28.35	184	5	19	5

Vegetables

Vegetable	Portion Size (g)	Calories	Protein (g)	Fiber (g)	Carbs (g)
Alfalfa Sprouts	30	9	2.3	1.2	1.7
Amaranth Leaves	30	7	1.5	1.7	2.1
Anaheim Pepper	150	7	1.2	1.5	2.4
Anise	15	24	2.2	3	4
Artichoke	150	65	4.5	8	15
Arugula	30	6	1.5	1.2	1.7
Asparagus	30	28	4	3.8	6
Avocado	50	81	2	4.4	5
Bamboo Shoots	30	14	2.2	2.8	3.5
Beet Greens	30	9	1.8	2.4	2.5
Beetroot	30	60	3.2	4.8	14
Bell Peppers	30	31	2	3.5	8
Bok Choy	30	10	2	2	2.5
Boston Lettuce	30	8	1.6	2	2.2
Broccoli	30	32	3.6	3.4	7
Brussels sprouts	30	39	4	4.3	9
Butterhead Lettuce	30	8	1.7	2	2.1
Cabbage	30	23	2.1	3.2	6
Carrot	150	26	1.6	2.7	7

Cauliflower	30	26	2.9	3	6
Celeriac	30	67	2.5	3.8	17
Celery	40	7	1.3	1.6	2.2
Chard	30	8	1.6	1.6	2.4
Chicory	30	8	1.1	1.9	2.4
Chives	30	20	3	3.5	3.7
Clover Sprouts	30	11	1.6	1.7	2
Collard Greens	30	12	2	2.4	3
Corn Salad	30	22	3	2.8	4.4
Cress	30	3	1.3	1.1	1.3
Cucumber	30	17	1.8	2	4.8
Daikon	30	23	1.6	2.6	6.2
Dandelion Greens	30	26	2.5	2.9	6
Dill	30	5	1.4	1.2	2
Dulse	30	19	1.2	3	5
Eggplant	30	21	1.8	3.5	6
Endive	30	9	1.6	2.7	2.7
Escarole	30	9	1.6	2.4	2.4
Fennel	30	28	2.1	3.7	7
Garlic	5	5	1.2	1.2	2
Green beans	30	32	3	4.4	8
Green Onion	15	6	1.1	1.4	2.3
Habanero Pepper	150	19	1.7	3.5	5.2
Horseradish	15	8	1.2	1.5	2.7
Jalapeño	150	5	1.1	1.4	1.9
Jalapeño	1 medium	5	1.1	1.4	1.9
Jerusalem Artichoke	1 cup	58	2.6	3.4	14.6
Jicama	1 cup	50	1.9	7.4	12
Jute Leaves	1 cup	7	1.9	1.9	2.1
Kale	1 cup	34	4	2	7
Kelp	1 cup	21	2.3	2	5

Kohlrabi	1 cup	37	3.3	5.9	9
Kohlrabi Greens	1 cup	19	2.5	2	4
Leeks	1 cup	33	1.6	2.6	9
Lettuce	1 cup	6	1.5	1.5	2
Lotus Root	1 cup	82	3.6	5.9	20
Mâche	1 cup	8	2	1.6	1.7
Mizuna	1 cup	11	2.3	1.9	2.5
Mung Bean Sprouts	1 cup	32	4.2	1.8	7
Mustard Greens	1 cup	16	2.6	3.8	3
Mustard Seeds	1 tbsp	53	3.1	4.3	3.1
Napa Cabbage	1 cup	21	2.2	2	5
Nori	1 sheet	6	2	1.5	2
Okra	1 cup	34	2.9	4.2	8
Onion	1 medium	45	2.3	2.9	11
Parsley	1 cup	23	2.8	3	4.8
Peas	1 cup	63	5	5.4	12
Pickles	1 medium	5	1.2	1.7	2.1
Poblano Pepper	1 medium	14	1.5	2.1	3.9
Purslane	1 cup	8	1.7	1.6	2.3
Radicchio	1 cup	10	1.2	1.9	2.8
Radish	1 cup	20	1.8	2.9	5
Rapini	1 cup	10	2.3	2.1	2.5
Rhubarb	1 cup	27	2.1	3.2	6.5
Romaine Lettuce	1 cup	9	1.6	2	2.5
Rutabaga	1 cup	53	2.5	4.2	13
Sauerkraut	1 cup	28	2.3	5	7
Scallions	1 medium	5.8	1.1	1.4	2.1
Seaweed	1 cup	31	3	1.3	8
Serrano Pepper	1 medium	2	1.1	1.1	1.2
Shallots	1 medium	8	1.3	1.4	2.7
Snow Peas	1 cup	27	2.6	2.6	5.9

Sorrel	1 cup	30	3.4	3.1	5
Spinach	1 cup	8	1.9	1.7	2.1
Squash	1 cup	19	1.4	2.2	5
Sweet Potato Leaf	1 cup	41	6	5	9
Swiss Chard	1 cup	8	1.6	1.6	2.4
Taro leaves	1 cup	43	2.5	4.7	10
Thai Chili	1 medium	2	1.1	1.1	1.2
Tomato	1 medium	23	2.1	2.5	5.8
Turnip	128	37	2.1	4.1	9
Wakame	128	21	2.1	1.3	5
Water Spinach	128	11	1.8	1.7	2.5
Watercress	128	5	1.8	1.2	1.4
Yardlong Beans	128	48	3.8	5	10
Yellow Pepper	120	51	2.7	3	12.8
Zucchini Flowers	128	6	1.5	1.5	2

Fruits

Fruit	Portion Size	Calories (kcal)	Carbohydrates (g)	Fiber (g)	Sugars (g)
Acai Berry	100 g	70	4	2	2
Acerola Cherry	1 cup (98g)	31	7.9	1.1	-
Apple	1 medium	95	25	4	19
Apricot	1 medium	17	3.9	0.7	3.2
Avocado	1 medium	322	17	13	1
Banana	1 medium	105	27	3	14
Black Currant	1 cup (112g)	71	17.2	5.4	13
Blackberry	1 cup	62	13.8	7.6	7
Blueberry	1 cup	84	21.4	3.6	14.7
Boysenberry	1 cup (144g)	61	14.7	7	10.9
Breadfruit	1 cup (220g)	227	59.7	10.8	29.7

Cactus Pear	1 fruit (103g)	42	9.9	3.7	5.9
Calamansi	100g	30	7.3	-	-
Camu Camu	100g	20	4.7	0.2	0.5
Cantaloupe	1 cup	53	13	1.4	12.3
Cape Gooseberry	1 cup (140g)	74	15.7	6	13.2
Cherimoya	1 cup (160g)	120	28.9	5.3	20.9
Cherry	1 cup	87	22	3	18
Cloudberry	100g	51	10.6	3.1	5.6
Cranberry	1 cup	46	12	4.6	4
Currant	1 cup	63	15.4	5.1	5
Date	1 medium	66	18	1.6	16
Dragon Fruit	1 cup	136	29	7	8
Durian	1 cup (243g)	357	65.8	9.2	44.3
Elderberry	1 cup	106	26.7	10.2	23
Feijoa	1 fruit (42g)	23	5.6	2.4	3.5
Fig	1 medium	37	9.6	1.4	8.1
Gac	100g	35	7	-	-
Grape	1 cup	62	16	0.8	15
Grapefruit	1 medium	52	13.1	2	8.5
Guava	1 medium	37	7.9	3	4.9
Hala Fruit	1 cup (250g)	140	36.3	5.3	20
Honeydew Melon	1 cup	64	16	1.4	14
Horned Melon	1 cup (233g)	103	24.5	2.9	13
Jabuticaba	1 cup (150g)	88	22.3	2.6	13.9
Jackfruit	1 cup	155	39.6	2.5	31.48
Jujube	1 cup (76g)	79	20.2	10	13.7
Kiwano (Horned Melon)	1 cup (233g)	103	24.5	2.9	13
Kiwi	1 medium	42	10.1	2.1	6.2
Kumquat	100 g	71	15.9	6.5	9.36
Langsat	1 cup (150g)	86	21.5	-	-

Lemon	1 medium	17	5.4	1.6	1.5
Lime	1 medium	20	7	1.9	1.1
Longan	1 cup (148g)	60	15.1	1.1	-
Loquat	1 cup (149g)	70	18.1	2.5	15.1
Lucuma	100g	92	21.3	2.3	14.6
Lychee	1 cup	125	31.4	2.5	28.9
Mamey Sapote	1 cup (175g)	215	56.3	9.5	34.2
Mango	1 cup	99	24.7	2.6	22.5
Mangosteen	1 cup (196g)	143	35.2	3.5	28.8
Maracuya (Passion Fruit)	1 fruit (18g)	17	4.2	2	2
Miracle Fruit	1 berry (2.5g)	1	0.2	0.1	0
Monk Fruit	100g	25	9.7	-	-
Mulberry	1 cup	60	13.7	2.4	11.3
Nance	1 cup (112g)	140	32	0.9	22
Nectarine	1 medium	63	15	2.4	11.2
Noni	1 fruit (100g)	47	10.4	3.1	-
Orange	1 medium	62	15.4	3.1	12.2
Papaya	1 cup	62	16	2.5	11
Papaya	1 cup	55	13.7	2.5	8.3
Passion Fruit	1 cup	229	55.2	24.5	26.4
Peach	1 medium	58	14	2	12
Pear	1 medium	102	27.5	5.5	17.4
Persimmon	1 medium	118	31.2	6	21
Pineapple	1 cup	82	21.6	2.3	16
Pitahaya (Dragon Fruit)	1 cup (227g)	136	29	7	8
Pitanga (Surinam Cherry)	1 cup (155g)	56	12.4	3.2	8.6
Plantain	1 medium (179g)	218	57	4	27.2
Plum	1 medium	30	7.5	1	6.6
Pomegranate	1 cup	144	32.5	7	24

Pomelo	1 cup (190g)	72	18.2	1.9	11.2
Prickly Pear	1 fruit (103g)	42	9.9	3.7	5.9
Quince	1 medium	52	14.1	1.9	0
Rambutan	1 cup	68	16.5	0.9	15.87
Rambutan	1 cup (150g)	68	16.5	0.9	15.87
Raspberry	1 cup	64	14.7	8	5.4
Red Currant	1 cup (112g)	63	15.4	4.6	7.37
Rose Apple	100g	25	5.7	1.5	4
Salak (Snake Fruit)	100g	82	20.9	2.8	8
Santol	100g	40	9.6	1.5	-
Sapodilla	1 fruit (170g)	199	48	9	35
Sea Buckthorn	100g	82	11	6	5
Soursop	1 cup	148	37.9	7.4	30.5
Soursop (Graviola)	1 cup (225g)	148	37.9	7.4	30.5
Star Apple	1 fruit (100g)	67	14.65	3	11
Starfruit	1 medium	28	6.2	2.8	3.6
Strawberry	1 cup	49	11.7	3	7.4
Strawberry Guava	100g	69	16	5.4	10
Sugar Apple (Sweetsop)	1 fruit (250g)	235	59.1	11.3	38
Tamarillo	1 fruit (100g)	31	3.9	3.3	3.2
Tamarind	1 cup (120g)	287	75	6.1	69
Tangerine	1 medium	47	11.7	1.6	9.3
Ugli fruit	1 medium	90	19	2	8
Velvet Apple	100g	81	19.1	1.2	13
Watermelon	1 cup	46	11.5	0.6	9.4
Wax Jambu (Water Apple)	100g	29	6.7	1.4	4.5
White Sapote	1 medium	135	34	5.3	23
Yellow Passion Fruit	1 fruit (18g)	17	4.2	2	2
Yuzu	100 g	52	15.9	1.7	0

Zucchini (yes, it's technically a fruit!)	1 cup	21	4.2	1.4	2.5

Legumes

Legumes	Portion Size (cooked)	Calories (kcal)	Protein (g)	Fiber (g)	Carbs (g)	Fat (g)
Adzuki beans	1 cup	294	17.3	16.8	57	0.2
Anasazi beans	1 cup	240	15.8	16.4	45.7	0.6
Azuki beans (Sweet red)	1 cup	294	17.3	16.8	57	0.2
Baked Beans	1 cup	239	12	10	54	0.9
Bambara beans	1 cup	200	11	6	35	1
Bean Burgers	1 patty	124	10	5	12	4.5
Bean Chips	1 oz (about 28g)	140	7	5	18	7
Bean Pasta	1 cup	200	14	8	35	1.5
Black Bean Brownies	1 brownie	112	2.5	3	24	1.5
Black Bean Soup	1 cup	227	15	15	40	1
Black beans	1 cup	227	15.2	15	41	0.9
Black lentils	1 cup	230	18	15.6	40	0.8
Black Turtle Beans	1 cup	227	15	15	41	0.9
Black-eyed peas	1 cup	160	5.2	8.2	35.5	0.6
Broad beans (Fava beans)	1 cup	187	13	9.2	33	0.7
Brown lentils	1 cup	230	18	15.6	40	0.8
Cannellini beans	1 cup	225	15	11	40.4	0.9
Chickpea flour (Besan)	1 cup	356	20.6	10.3	53	6.2
Chickpea Pasta	1 cup	190	14	8	32	3.5

Chickpea Salad	1 cup	269	14.5	12.5	45	4.2
Chickpeas (Garbanzo beans)	1 cup	269	14.5	12.5	45	4.2
Cowpeas	1 cup	160	5.2	8.2	35.5	0.6
Cranberry beans	1 cup	241	16.5	17.7	43.4	0.9
Dal Makhani (Mixed Lentils and Beans)	1 cup	230	12	15	30	10
Edamame	1 cup	189	17	8	13.8	8
Edamame Hummus	1 cup	180	8	5	14	10
Egyptian White Beans	1 cup	240	17	12	43	1.2
Ethiopian Berbere Beans	1 cup	210	13	16	39	1
Ethiopian Teff (used in traditional injera)	1 cup	255	9.8	5	50	1.5
Fava beans	1 cup	187	13	9.2	33	0.7
Fermented Black Beans (Douchi)	1 cup	220	19	16	35	2
Flageolet Beans	1 cup	229	13.4	9.0	33.5	0.8
French Green Lentils	1 cup	230	17.9	15.6	39.9	0.8
French lentils (Puy)	1 cup	230	17.9	15.6	39.9	0.8
Garbanzo beans (Chickpeas)	1 cup	269	14.5	12.5	45	4.2
Great Northern beans	1 cup	209	14.7	12.4	37.3	0.7
Greek Gigantes Beans	1 cup	198	13.2	9.5	35.7	0.8

Green beans	1 cup	44	2.4	3.7	10	0.3
Green lentils	1 cup	230	18	15.6	40	0.8
Hummus (Chickpea Paste)	1 cup	408	19	15	35	24
Hyacinth beans	1 cup	227	15.3	11.1	40.4	0.9
Indian Chana Dal (Split Chickpeas)	1 cup	269	14.5	12.5	45	4.2
Indian Masoor Dal (Red Lentils)	1 cup	230	17.9	15.6	39.9	0.8
Indian Rajma (Kidney Beans)	1 cup	225	15	11	40	0.9
Indian Toor Dal (Pigeon Peas)	1 cup	209	11.1	8	39	0.8
Indian Urad Dal (Black Lentils)	1 cup	230	18	15.6	40	0.8
Italian Borlotti Beans	1 cup	240	17	13	46	0.6
Japanese Azuki Beans	1 cup	294	17.3	16.8	57	0.2
Kidney beans	1 cup	225	15.3	11.3	40.4	0.9
Lentil Chips	1 oz (about 28g)	110	3	1	19	4
Lentil Curry	1 cup	240	9	15	35	10
Lentil Soup	1 cup	186	11	8	30	2
Lentils	1 cup	230	18	15.6	40	0.8
Lima beans	1 cup	216	14.7	13.2	39.3	0.7
Lupin Beans	1 cup	200	26	4.6	16	4.8
Lupini beans	1 cup	198	26	4.6	16	4.8
Mexican Bayo Beans	1 cup	215	14	9	38	0.9
Moth beans	1 cup	200	14.5	8	35.5	1.1
Mung beans	1 cup	212	14.2	15.4	38.7	0.8

Mung dal (Yellow split)	1 cup	212	14.2	15.4	38.7	0.8
Navy beans	1 cup	255	15	19.1	47.5	1.1
Navy beans	1 cup	255	15	19.1	47.5	1.1
Northern beans	1 cup	209	14.7	12.4	37.3	0.7
Pea Protein Milk	1 cup	70	8	2	0	4.5
Pea Soup	1 cup	185	11	4.5	34	1
Peanut (Raw)	1 cup	828	38	12	24	72
Peanut Butter	2 tbsp	188	8	2	6	16
Peanut Sauce	2 tbsp	70	2	1	3	6
Peas	1 cup	117	7.9	7.4	21	0.6
Peruvian Canary Beans	1 cup	225	14.5	10.5	40.2	0.6
Pigeon peas	1 cup	209	11.1	8.0	39.0	0.8
Pinto beans	1 cup	245	15.4	15.4	44.8	1.1
Red Bean Paste	1 cup	240	7	4	55	0.5
Red lentils	1 cup	230	17.9	15.6	39.9	0.8
Refried Beans	1 cup	237	13	10	35	3
Roman beans	1 cup	225	15.3	11.3	40.4	0.9
Rosecoco beans	1 cup	217	14.5	13.1	39.6	0.8
Salted Soybeans (Natto)	1 cup	185	18	5	14	11
Scarlet runner beans	1 cup	225	15.2	11.3	40.4	0.9
Small red beans	1 cup	218	16.5	13.1	39.7	0.6
Soy Ice Cream	1 cup	210	4	3	24	12
Soy Milk	1 cup	131	8	1	15	4
Soy Protein Powder	1 scoop	95	20	1	2	1.5
Soy Yogurt	1 cup	150	6	2	16	4
Soybean Oil	1 tbsp	120	0	0	0	14

Soybean Sprouts	1 cup	85	9	3	6	4.5
Soybeans	1 cup	298	28.6	10.3	17.1	15.4
Spanish Tolosana Beans	1 cup	225	15.2	12.4	40.5	0.5
Split peas	1 cup	231	16.3	16.3	41.4	0.8
Sprouted Black Beans	1 cup	90	6.2	8.4	15.2	0.5
Sprouted Chickpeas	1 cup	120	11	9.6	22	2
Sprouted Lentils	1 cup	82	6.9	7.8	17.1	0.4
Sprouted Mung Beans	1 cup	31	3.2	0.8	6.2	0.2
Tempeh	1 cup	320	31	7	16	18
Tepary beans	1 cup	215	15	15	39	1
Turkish Fasulye Beans	1 cup	220	14	11	38	0.7
Velvet beans	1 cup	220	15	10	35	1.5
White beans	1 cup	249	17	11.3	45.5	0.6
Winged beans	1 cup	241	18.3	16.3	43.5	0.9

Dairy or Dairy Alternatives

Dairy or Dairy Alternatives	Portion Size	Calories (kcal)	Protein (g)	Fat (g)	Carbohydrates (g)
A2 Cow's Milk	1 cup	148	8	8	12
Almond Cheese (unsweetened)	1 oz	70	3	6	1
Almond Milk (unsweetened)	1 cup	30	1	2.5	1
Almond Milk Creamer (unsweetened)	1 tbsp	10	0	1	0

Almond Yogurt (unsweetened)	100g	40	1.5	2.5	2
Blue Cheese	1 oz	100	6	8	1
Brie Cheese	1 oz	95	6	8	0.1
Buffalo Milk	1 cup	237	9	17	13
Butter (grass-fed)	1 tbsp	102	0.1	11.5	0
Camel Milk	1 cup	107	5.4	4.6	8
Camembert Cheese	1 oz	85	5	7	0.1
Casein Protein Powder (unsweetened)	1 scoop	120	24	1	3
Cashew Milk (unsweetened)	1 cup	25	0	2	1
Cashew Yogurt (unsweetened)	100g	120	3	9	8
Chia Milk (unsweetened)	1 cup	70	2	4	1
Coconut Cream (unsweetened)	1 tbsp	50	0.5	5	1
Coconut Milk (light, canned)	1 cup	445	4.6	48	6.4
Coconut Milk Yogurt (unsweetened)	100g	150	1	12	8
Coconut Yogurt (unsweetened)	100g	150	2	12	8
Cream Cheese (low-fat)	1 oz	29	3.5	2.5	1.1
Edam Cheese	1 oz	101	7	8	1
Emmental Cheese	1 oz	113	8	9	0.1
Ewe's Milk Cheese	1 oz	100	7	8	1
Feta Cheese	1 oz	75	4	6	1.2
Flax Milk (unsweetened)	1 cup	25	0	2.5	1
Ghee (clarified butter)	1 tbsp	112	0	12.8	0
Goat Cheese	1 oz	75	5	6	0.1
Goat Milk Kefir	1 cup	162	9	10	11

Goat's Milk Cheese (soft)	1 oz	75	5	6	0.1
Gouda Cheese	1 oz	101	7	8	0.6
Greek Yogurt (full-fat)	100g	97	9	5	4
Halloumi Cheese	1 oz	110	7	9	1
Hard Cheese (Cheddar)	1 oz	113	7	9	0.4
Hazelnut Milk (unsweetened)	1 cup	30	1	3.5	1
Hemp Milk (unsweetened)	1 cup	60	3	4.5	0
Kefir (low-fat)	1 cup	104	11	2	12
Lactose-Free Cheese (hard)	1 oz	110	7	9	0
Lactose-Free Ice Cream	1/2 cup	160	3	9	19
Lactose-Free Milk (skim)	1 cup	90	8	0	13
Lactose-Free Yogurt (plain)	100g	56	5.7	0.4	7.8
Low-fat Cottage Cheese	100g	98	11	2.3	3.4
Low-fat Greek Yogurt	100g	59	10	0.4	3.6
Macadamia Milk (unsweetened)	1 cup	50	1	5	1
Mascarpone	1 tbsp	120	1.5	12	1
Mozzarella (part-skim)	1 oz	72	6.3	4.5	0.9
Nutritional Yeast	2 tbsp	45	8	0.5	5
Nutritional Yeast (fortified)	2 tbsp	60	8	1	5
Oat Milk (unsweetened)	1 cup	120	3	5	16
Oat Yogurt (unsweetened)	100g	90	4	4	12
Paneer (cottage cheese)	100g	265	18	20	1.2

Pea Protein Milk (unsweetened)	1 cup	70	8	4.5	0
Pea Yogurt (unsweetened)	100g	100	6	5	5
Provolone Cheese	1 oz	100	7	8	0.6
Quark (low-fat)	100g	74	14	0.3	3.9
Rice Milk (unsweetened)	1 cup	113	0.7	2.3	22
Ricotta Cheese (part-skim)	1/4 cup	85	7	5	3
Sheep Milk	1 cup	265	14	17	13
Skim Milk	1 cup	83	8	0.2	12
Skyr (Icelandic yogurt, plain)	100g	61	11	0.2	4
Sour Cream (light)	1 tbsp	20	0.3	1.7	0.6
Soy Cheese	1 oz	80	7	5	2
Soy Cream Cheese	1 oz	80	2	7	2
Soy Milk	1 cup	105	6	4.3	12
Soy Milk Powder	1 tbsp	35	3	1.5	2
Soy Yogurt (unsweetened)	100g	94	4	4	7
Tempeh	100g	193	19	11	9
Tofu (firm, calcium-set)	100g	144	17	9	2
Unsweetened Whey Protein	1 scoop	110	24	1	2
Vegan Butter	1 tbsp	100	0	11	0
Vegan Cheddar Cheese	1 oz	90	0	7	9
Vegan Cheese Spread	1 tbsp	45	0	4.5	1
Vegan Cottage Cheese	1/2 cup	90	1	5	6
Vegan Cream Cheese	1 oz	80	1	8	4
Vegan Greek Yogurt (unsweetened)	100g	59	4	2	3.5
Vegan Ice Cream (almond milk-based)	1/2 cup	180	2	9	21

Vegan Ice Cream (cashew milk-based)	1/2 cup	160	3	9	18
Vegan Ice Cream (coconut-based)	1/2 cup	200	2	12	22
Vegan Ice Cream (oat milk-based)	1/2 cup	140	2	7	21
Vegan Ice Cream (soy milk-based)	1/2 cup	150	2	7	24
Vegan Kefir (almond-based)	1 cup	60	1	3	8
Vegan Kefir (cashew-based)	1 cup	90	2	6	9
Vegan Kefir (coconut-based)	1 cup	70	1	5	7
Vegan Kefir (soy-based)	1 cup	80	6	4	6
Vegan Mozzarella Cheese	1 oz	85	0	6	7
Vegan Parmesan Cheese	2 tbsp	20	2	1.5	2
Vegan Protein Powder (hemp-based)	1 scoop	110	15	3	9
Vegan Protein Powder (pea-based)	1 scoop	120	24	2	3
Vegan Protein Powder (rice-based)	1 scoop	120	24	1	4
Vegan Protein Powder (soy-based)	1 scoop	110	25	1	2
Vegan Protein Shake (pre-made)	1 bottle	160	20	3	9
Vegan Ricotta Cheese	1/4 cup	100	5	8	5
Vegan Sour Cream	1 tbsp	35	0.5	3	2
Vegan Yogurt (almond-based)	100g	60	2	3	8
Vegan Yogurt (cashew-based)	100g	120	3	9	8

Vegan Yogurt (coconut-based)	100g	150	1	12	8
Vegan Yogurt (oat-based)	100g	70	1	2	12
Vegan Yogurt (pea protein-based)	100g	70	6	2	8
Vegan Yogurt (soy-based)	100g	95	6	4	7
Yogurt (plant-based, unsweetened)	100g	59	4	3	6

Herbs and Spices

Spices	Portion Size	Calories (kcal)	Carbs (g)	Protein (g)	Fat (g)
Turmeric	1 tsp	9	2.1	0.3	0.1
Cinnamon	1 tsp	6	2.1	0.1	0.1
Ginger	1 tsp	2	0.4	0.0	0.0
Cayenne Pepper	1 tsp	6	1.0	0.2	0.3
Black Pepper	1 tsp	5	1.3	0.2	0.1
Cumin	1 tsp	8	0.9	0.4	0.5
Cardamom	1 tsp	6	1.4	0.2	0.1
Clove	1 tsp	6	1.3	0.1	0.3
Nutmeg	1 tsp	12	1.1	0.1	0.8
Paprika	1 tsp	6	1.2	0.3	0.3
Rosemary	1 tsp	4	0.6	0.1	0.2
Thyme	1 tsp	3	0.7	0.1	0.1
Oregano	1 tsp	5	1.0	0.1	0.1
Basil	1 tsp	1	0.1	0.1	0.0
Parsley	1 tbsp	1	0.2	0.1	0.0

Whole Food Snacks

Whole Food Snack	Portion Size	Calories (approx.)	Protein (g)	Fats (g)	Carbohydrates (g)
Air-Popped Popcorn	3 cups (24g)	90	3	1	18
Almond Yogurt with Cinnamon	1 cup (245g)	180	5	9	20
Almonds	1 oz (28g)	160	6	14	6
Apple Slices with Almond Butter	1 apple + 1 tbsp (16g) butter	200	2	11	25
Avocado	1/2 medium	130	2	12	7
Baked Cod with Lemon	3 oz (85g)	70	15	1	0
Baked Kale and Spinach Balls	4 balls	100	5	7	10
Baked Sweet Potato Chips	1 cup (35g)	150	2	5	24
Beef Biltong	1 oz (28g)	80	16	2	0
Bell Pepper Slices with Ranch	1 bell pepper + 2 tbsp (30g) ranch	150	1	14	9
Berries (mixed)	1 cup (144g)	70	1	0.5	17
Blueberries with Greek Yogurt	1/2 cup berries + 1/2 cup yogurt	120	12	0.5	18
Brazil Nuts	1 oz (28g)	185	4	18	3
Caprese Skewers	3 skewers	150	9	10	6
Carrot Sticks with Hummus	10 sticks + 2 tbsp (30g) hummus	100	3	5.5	11.5
Celery Sticks with Peanut Butter	2 sticks + 1 tbsp (16g) butter	100	4	8	3
Cherry Tomatoes with Mozzarella	5 tomatoes + 1 oz (28g) cheese	100	8	6	3

Chia Seed Pudding	1/2 cup (120g)	150	4	9	13
Cottage Cheese (low-fat)	1 cup (226g)	160	28	2.3	6.2
Cottage Cheese and Pineapple	1/2 cup (113g) cottage cheese + 1/2 cup pineapple	150	15	2	20
Cottage Cheese with Berries	1/2 cup (113g) + 1/2 cup berries	120	14	0.5	18
Cucumber and Feta Cheese Salad	1 cup	104	6	7	3.5
Edamame	1 cup (155g)	190	17	8	16
Greek Salad Bites	5 bites	150	5	12	7
Greek Yogurt (plain, low-fat)	1 cup (245g)	130	23	3	10
Greek Yogurt with Chia Seeds	1 cup (245g) yogurt + 1 tbsp chia	190	24	4	15
Grilled Chicken Strips	3 oz (85g)	130	25	3	0
Grilled Zucchini with Parmesan	1 medium zucchini + 1 tbsp Parmesan	100	7	7	4
Guacamole with Jicama Sticks	1/4 cup guacamole + 1/2 cup sticks	120	2	9	10
Hard-Boiled Egg Whites	4 egg whites	68	14	0	0.6
Hard-Boiled Eggs	2 eggs	140	12	10	1
Kale Chips	1 cup (20g)	74	2.2	4.9	7.3
Kiwi Slices	1 cup (180g)	110	2	1	26
Mixed Nuts	1 oz (28g)	170	5	15	6
Mixed Vegetable Sticks	1 cup	50	1.5	0.3	11
Olives	1 oz (28g)	40	0	4	1

Pear Slices with Ricotta Cheese	1 pear + 1/4 cup (62g) ricotta	150	5	7	22
Protein Smoothie (whey protein)	1 serving	200	20	3	10
Pumpkin Seeds	1 oz (28g)	150	7	13	5
Quinoa Salad with Veggies	1 cup (185g)	222	8	3.6	39.4
Raw Veggie Salad with Lemon Juice	2 cups mixed veggies	100	2	5	18
Roasted Brussels Sprouts	1 cup (88g)	56	4	0.8	11
Roasted Chickpeas	1/2 cup (82g)	130	6	2	22
Sardines in Olive Oil	1 can (92g)	190	23	10	0
Seaweed Snacks	1 package (5g)	25	2	2	1
Shrimp Cocktail	3 oz (85g) shrimp	100	20	1.5	2
Sliced Avocado and Tomato	1/2 avocado + 1/2 tomato	150	2	13	8
Sliced Cucumber with Guacamole	1/2 cup sliced + 2 tbsp (30g) guac	80	1	6	4
Sliced Peaches with Cottage Cheese	1 cup sliced + 1/2 cup (113g) cheese	150	14	0.5	25
Smoked Salmon on Cucumber Slices	2 oz (56g) salmon + cucumber	100	12	4	1
Smoked Turkey Roll-ups	3 oz (85g) turkey	90	18	1	2
Snap Peas with Tahini	1 cup snap peas + 1 tbsp (15g) tahini	100	5	8	10
Spiced Pumpkin Seeds	1 oz (28g)	153	7	13	5
Spinach and Feta Stuffed Mushrooms	4 mushrooms	100	6	7	4

Steamed Edamame with Sea Salt	1 cup (155g)	188	18	8	14
String Cheese	1 piece (28g)	80	7	5	1
Sunflower Seeds	1 oz (28g)	160	6	14	6
Tofu Stir Fry with Broccoli	1 cup	150	12	9	10
Tuna Salad on Bell Pepper	1/2 cup (100g) tuna salad + bell pepper	150	20	7	4
Turkey Jerky	1 oz (28g)	80	11	1	6
Walnuts	1 oz (28g)	180	4	18	4
Watermelon Slices	1 cup (152g)	46	0.9	0.2	11.6
Zucchini Chips	1 cup (85g)	100	1	7	8

FOODS TO AVOID

Refined Carbohydrates

Refined Carbohydrates	Portion Size	Calories (approx.)	Carbs (g)	Sugars (g)	Fiber (g)	Protein (g)
Baguette	1/4 loaf	185	36	1	2	6
Breakfast pastries	1 pastry	410	50	20	1	5
Cake	1 slice	235	34	24	0.5	3
Candy bars	1 bar	250	33	28	1	3
Chocolate	1 oz	150	17	15	1	2
Cookies	2 medium	160	20	12	0.5	2
Corn flakes	1 cup	100	24	2	1	2
Corn syrup	2 tbsp	120	30	30	0	0
Croissants	1 medium	235	26	6	1.5	5
Doughnuts	1 medium	250	31	15	1	4
Energy drinks	8 oz	110	28	27	0	0
Flavored gelatin	1/2 cup	80	19	19	0	2
French fries	3 oz	230	29	0	3	3
Fruit canned in heavy syrup	1/2 cup	100	26	23	0.5	0
Fruit-flavored yogurt	6 oz	150	26	19	0	6
Granola bars	1 bar	120	18	8	2	3
Honey	1 tbsp	64	17	17	0	0.1
Ice cream	1/2 cup	140	17	14	0	2
Instant oatmeal (flavored)	1 packet	150	27	12	3	4
Maple syrup	2 tbsp	104	27	24	0	0
Muffins	1 medium	300	45	24	1	5
Pancakes	2 pancakes	200	38	8	1	6
Pies	1 slice	277	42	18	2	3
Popcorn (buttered)	3 cups	170	19	0	3	2

Potato chips	1 oz	160	15	1	1	2
Pretzels	1 oz	108	22	1	1	2.8
Pudding	1/2 cup	140	26	20	0	3
Regular pasta	1 cup cooked	220	43	2	2.5	8
Rice cakes	1 cake	35	7	0	0	1
Soda	12 oz can	150	39	39	0	0
Soft drinks	12 oz	150	39	39	0	0
Sports drinks	8 oz	50	14	10	0	0
Sugar-sweetened beverages	12 oz	140	35	35	0	0
Sweet rolls	1 roll	223	30	16	1	4
Sweetened condensed milk	1 oz	123	21	21	0	3
Tortilla chips	1 oz	140	18	0	1	2
Waffles	2 waffles	220	30	6	1	5
White bagel	1 medium	250	50	5	2	9
White bread	1 slice	70	15	2	1	2
White crackers	5 crackers	80	10	0	0	1
White rice	1 cup cooked	200	45	0	0.6	4
White sugar	1 tsp	16	4.2	4.2	0	0

Sugary Snacks and Beverages

Sugary Snacks and Beverages	Portion Size	Calories (approx.)	Carbohydrates (g)	Sugars (g)	Fat (g)	Sodium (mg)
Biscotti	1 biscotti	110	16	10	4	95
Brownies	1 square	130	18	15	6	65
Bubble tea	16 oz	200	50	38	0	100
Candy bars	1 bar	250	33	27	14	120
Candy gummies	10 pieces	200	46	29	0	15

Caramel macchiato	16 oz	250	33	32	7	150
Cereal bars	1 bar	130	24	8	3	90
Cheesecake	1 slice	257	20	18	18	175
Chocolate bar	1.55 oz	220	28	24	13	35
Chocolate milkshake	12 oz	530	68	63	15	240
Chocolate pudding	1/2 cup	160	26	19	7	210
Cookies	2 cookies	160	25	14	8	140
Cupcakes	1 cupcake	195	29	24	9	160
Doughnut	1 medium	250	31	15	14	190
Energy drinks	8 oz	110	28	27	0	150
Flavored coffee creamer	1 tbsp	35	5	5	1.5	15
Flavored gelatin	1/2 cup	80	19	18	0	55
Flavored milk	8 oz	210	26	24	8	130
Frosted pastries	1 pastry	420	75	24	10	340
Fruit cocktail in syrup	1/2 cup	110	28	23	0	10
Fruit pie	1 slice	300	58	25	12	400
Fruit punch	8 oz	120	29	28	0	20
Fruit smoothie	12 oz	250	62	47	0	30
Fruit-flavored yogurt	6 oz	150	26	19	2	85
Gelato	1/2 cup	160	25	20	7	40
Granola bars	1 bar	140	19	11	6	95
Honey	1 tbsp	64	17	17	0	1
Ice cream	1/2 cup	137	16	14	7	53
Jam or jelly	1 tbsp	56	14	14	0	6
Lattes (flavored)	16 oz	190	18	17	7	95
Lemonade	8 oz	99	26	25	0	5
Maple syrup	2 tbsp	104	27	24	0	7
Marshmallows	4 large	90	22	15	0	25
Milk chocolate	1 oz	150	13	12	8	20

Mocha coffee	16 oz	330	43	25	15	120
Muffins	1 medium	340	50	20	10	400
Pancake syrup	2 tbsp	110	28	24	0	75
Pastries (Danish)	1 Danish	263	31	17	14	200
Popsicles	1 popsicle	80	20	14	0	0
Soda	12 oz	150	39	39	0	10
Sorbet	1/2 cup	100	25	24	0	5
Sports drinks	12 oz	90	21	20	0	150
Sweet potato fries	1 cup	160	34	7	4	170
Sweetened cereal	1 cup	160	37	17	1	200
Sweetened condensed milk	1 tbsp	61	10	10	1.5	22
Sweetened iced tea	12 oz	140	36	35	0	10
Sweetened popcorn	1 bag	300	50	25	15	500
Sweetened whipped cream	2 tbsp	52	4	4	4.5	1
Tiramisu	1 slice	240	30	17	11	85
Waffles (frozen, sweetened)	2 waffles	180	30	6	6	360

Processed Foods

Processed Food	Portion Size	Calories (kcal)	Carbs (g)	Sugars (g)	Fats (g)	Saturated Fats (g)	Sodium (mg)
Bagels	1 bagel	245	48	6	1.5	0.3	450
BBQ Sauce	2 tbsp (30ml)	60	14	12	0	0	280
Bottled Frappuccino	13.7 oz (405ml)	290	45	43	4.5	2.5	115
Bottled Smoothies	8 oz (240ml)	130	31	29	0	0	25

Boxed Cake Mix	1/10 package	280	53	35	4	2	380
Breakfast Cereals (Sweetened)	1 cup (30g)	120	24	11	1.5	0.3	200
Cake	1 slice	235	34	24	10	3	210
Candy	1 oz (28g)	113	28	21	0	0	5
Canned Baked Beans in Sauce	1/2 cup	190	36	12	0.5	0	570
Canned Chili with Beans	1 cup	287	30	4	14	6	890
Canned Fruit in Syrup	1/2 cup	100	26	23	0	0	10
Canned Soup (Cream-based)	1 cup (245g)	200	15	5	13	5	800
Canned Spaghetti Sauce	1/2 cup	70	13	9	2	0.3	460
Cereal Bars	1 bar	130	24	12	3	0.5	200
Chocolate Bar	1 bar (42g)	220	25	20	14	8	35
Chocolate Syrup	2 tbsp	100	24	20	0	0	35
Cookies	2 cookies	140	20	12	6	2.5	90

Cream Cheese Frosting	2 tbsp	140	20	18	6	4	70
Doughnuts	1 doughnut	250	31	17	12	6	320
Energy Drinks	8 oz (240 ml)	110	28	27	0	0	150
Fast Food Burger	1 burger	540	40	10	30	10	940
Flavored Coffee Creamer	1 tbsp	35	5	5	1.5	1	10
Flavored Gelatin	1/2 cup	80	19	19	0	0	55
Flavored Instant Oatmeal	1 packet	150	27	12	2	0.5	240
Flavored Milk	8 oz (240 ml)	150	18	17	2.5	1.5	100
Flavored Potato Crisps	1 oz (28g)	160	15	2	10	3	180
Flavored Protein Bars	1 bar	220	20	15	9	5	320
Flavored Rice Mix	1 cup prepared	210	44	1	0.5	0	750
Flavored Tofu	3 oz (85g)	70	2	1	4	0.5	15
Flavored Water (Sweetened)	16.9 oz (500ml)	120	30	30	0	0	20

Flavored Yogurt	1 cup (245g)	230	47	44	3	2	150
French Fries	1 small	230	29	0	11	2	160
Fried Chicken	1 piece	320	8	0	24	3.5	690
Frozen Fish Sticks	4 sticks	230	24	1	10	2	530
Frozen Meat Pies	1 pie	480	35	1	30	15	850
Frozen Pizza	1/4 pizza	320	35	4	14	5	720
Frozen Waffles	2 waffles	220	30	6	9	2	460
Fruit Snacks	1 pouch (23g)	80	19	11	0	0	10
Ice Cream	1/2 cup (68g)	137	16	14	7	4.5	53
Instant Mac & Cheese	1 cup (prepared)	220	27	3	9	3	470
Instant Noodles	1 package	380	51	2	14	6	1580
Instant Pudding	1/2 cup prepared	90	23	19	0	0	350
Margarine	1 tbsp (14g)	100	0	0	11	2	150
Microwave Popcorn	1 bag	400	40	0	20	12	500
Packaged Cupcakes	1 cupcake	180	27	18	7	1.5	150
Packaged Granola	1/2 cup	200	32	12	7	2	100

Packaged Pastries	1 pastry	410	45	24	24	12	360
Packaged Snack Cakes	1 cake	270	45	30	9	2.5	380
Potato Chips	1 oz (28g)	155	14	1	10	3	170
Pre-made Pie Crust	1/8 crust	80	10	1	5	2.5	110
Pre-made Salad Dressing	2 tbsp	140	2	1	15	2.5	260
Pre-packaged Sushi Rolls	1 package	350	71	10	3	0.5	800
Pre-sliced Fruit Loaf	1 slice	90	18	8	1	0.2	125
Processed Cheese	1 slice (21g)	70	1	0	6	3.5	350
Processed Deli Sandwich	1 sandwich	600	50	5	30	10	1260
Processed Meat (e.g., Salami)	2 slices	190	1	0	17	6	620
Processed Vegan Cheese	1 oz (28g)	80	7	0	6	5	280
Soda	12 oz (355 ml)	150	39	39	0	0	10
Sports Drinks	8 oz (240 ml)	50	14	10	0	0	100

Sweetened Almond Milk	8 oz (240ml)	60	8	7	2.5	0	150
Sweetened Condensed Milk	1 tbsp	61	10	10	1.5	1	22
Sweetened Dried Fruit	1/4 cup	100	25	20	0	0	2
Sweetened Iced Tea	8 oz (240 ml)	90	22	22	0	0	10
White Bread	1 slice (28g)	75	14	2	1	0.2	150

High-Fat Meats

High-Fat Meats	Portion Size	Calories (approx.)	Total Fat (g)	Saturated Fat (g)	Cholesterol (mg)	Protein (g)
Andouille Sausage	2 oz	170	14	5	50	10
Bacon	2 slices	70	7	3	15	4
Bacon	2 slices	70	7	3	15	4
Beef Jerky	1 oz	116	7	3	40	9
Beef Jerky	1 oz	116	7	3	40	9
Beef Short Ribs	3 oz	210	14	6	70	24
Bison Ribeye	3 oz	190	10	4	55	24
Bologna (Beef)	1 slice	90	8	3	20	3
Bologna (Beef)	1 slice	90	8	3	20	3
Brisket (Beef)	3 oz	210	13	5	60	24

Brisket (Beef)	3 oz	210	13	5	60	24
Capicola	1 oz	80	5	2	20	7
Chicken Wings (Fried)	3 wings	220	15	4	75	20
Chicken Wings (Fried)	3 wings	220	15	4	75	20
Chorizo	1 oz	129	11	4	25	7
Chorizo	1 oz	129	11	4	25	7
Corned Beef	3 oz	210	16	5	90	15
Corned Beef	3 oz	210	16	5	90	15
Duck Breast	3 oz	200	11	4	85	23
Duck Breast	3 oz	200	11	4	85	23
Duck Confit	3 oz	275	23	8	105	16
Duck Confit	3 oz	275	23	8	105	16
Elk Meat	3 oz	160	7	3	60	22
Fatty Fish (e.g., Salmon)	3 oz	200	12	3	60	23
Foie Gras	1 oz	110	10	4	85	4
Goose	3 oz	340	29	11	85	22
Goose	3 oz	340	29	11	85	22
Ground Beef (80/20)	3 oz	230	15	6	75	22
Ground Beef (80/20)	3 oz	230	15	6	75	22
Kielbasa	2 oz	180	15	5	40	8
Lamb Chop	3 oz	250	21	9	85	19
Lamb Shoulder	3 oz	250	21	9	85	17
Lamb Shoulder	3 oz	250	21	9	85	17

Lardo	1 oz	115	12	5	25	0
Mortadella	1 oz	90	8	3	20	5
Pate (Liver)	1 oz	100	8	3	95	6
Pate (Liver)	1 oz	100	8	3	95	6
Pepperoni	1 oz	140	13	5	35	6
Pepperoni	1 oz	140	13	5	35	6
Pheasant	3 oz	190	8	3	90	25
Pork Belly	3 oz	330	30	11	90	9
Pork Belly	3 oz	330	30	11	90	9
Pork Chop (Bone-in)	3 oz	250	20	7	75	23
Pork Ribs (Baby Back)	3 oz	250	20	7	80	20
Pork Ribs (Baby Back)	3 oz	250	20	7	80	20
Prosciutto	1 oz	70	5	2	20	10
Quail	1 whole	123	4.2	1.2	64	21.8
Rabbit	3 oz	170	7	2	70	28
Ribeye Steak	3 oz	250	20	9	75	20
Ribeye Steak	3 oz	250	20	9	75	20
Salami	1 oz	110	9	3	30	7
Salami	1 oz	110	9	3	30	7
Sausage (Pork)	2 links	170	15	5	40	7
Sausage (Pork)	2 links	170	15	5	40	7
Smoked Turkey Leg	3 oz	200	11	3	90	28
Speck	1 oz	100	8	3	20	7
T-bone Steak	3 oz	210	14	6	70	20
T-bone Steak	3 oz	210	14	6	70	20

Turkey Bacon	2 slices	70	5	1.5	30	5
Turkey Sausage	2 links	140	9	2.5	60	14
Veal Rib	3 oz	230	16	7	80	22
Venison (Deer Meat)	3 oz	180	8	4	90	26
Wild Boar	3 oz	210	13	5	80	22

High-Sodium Snacks

High-Sodium Snacks	Portion Size	Calories (approx.)	Sodium (mg)	Carbohydrates (g)	Protein (g)	Fat (g)
Pretzels	1 oz (28g)	108	385	22.5	2.6	0.8
Salted Peanuts	1 oz (28g)	166	230	4.6	6.7	14.1
Potato Chips	1 oz (28g)	155	170	14.1	2.0	10.5
Instant Noodles	1 package	380	1580	51	9	14
Cheese Puffs	1 oz (28g)	155	240	9.1	1.9	10.5
Salted Popcorn	1 oz (28g)	155	325	18.1	5	9.5
Soy Sauce (for dipping)	1 tbsp	11	902	1	2	0
Pickles	1 medium	12	833	2.7	0.3	0.2
Anchovies	1 oz (28g)	42	1176	0	5.8	1.9
Beef Jerky	1 oz (28g)	116	506	3.1	9.4	7.3
Canned Soup	1 cup	150	940	18.3	7.9	5.0
Ramen Noodles	1 package	380	1820	54	10	14
Salted Cashews	1 oz (28g)	157	12	9.2	5.1	12.3
Frozen Pizza	1 slice	285	640	33	12	10
Olives	1 oz (28g)	41	735	1.1	0.3	4.3
Salted Almonds	1 oz (28g)	169	96	6.1	6.0	14.9
Sardines in Oil	1 can	191	465	0	22.7	10.5
Hot Dogs	1 hot dog	151	560	2	5	13
Bacon	2 slices	106	450	0.3	7	7.9

Salted Pistachios	1 oz (28g)	158	121	7.7	5.8	12.6
Deli Meats	1 oz (28g)	37	360	1	5.5	1
Cheese Crackers	1 oz (28g)	142	211	19	2.9	7
Salted Sunflower Seeds	1 oz (28g)	164	174	6.8	5.8	14
Canned Chili	1 cup	287	1309	30.2	14.7	15.3
Nacho Cheese Dip	1 oz (28g)	60	240	5	2	4
Salted Macadamia Nuts	1 oz (28g)	204	1	3.9	2.2	21.5
Caesar Salad (fast food)	1 serving	184	400	10.3	7.1	12.9
Spicy Chicken Wings	3 wings	216	870	0	18.4	15.5
Instant Mashed Potatoes	1 cup	237	800	37	4	1
Corned Beef	3 oz (85g)	213	827	0.4	15.5	16.2
Salted Pretzel Sticks	1 oz (28g)	108	385	22.5	2.6	0.8
Smoked Salmon	2 oz (56g)	70	666	0	11.9	1.4
Salted Bagel Chips	1 oz (28g)	130	210	20	3	4
Tortilla Chips	1 oz (28g)	140	115	19	2	7
Salted Pumpkin Seeds	1 oz (28g)	153	92	5	7	13
Microwave Popcorn	1 oz (28g)	151	300	10	3	10
Salted Sesame Sticks	1 oz (28g)	160	190	14	4	10

Chicken Nuggets (fast food)	6 pieces	270	540	18	14	16
French Fries (fast food)	Medium	365	246	48	4	17
Onion Rings (fast food)	Medium	411	820	58	5	18
Salted Mixed Nuts	1 oz (28g)	170	120	5	5	15
Queso Dip	1 oz (28g)	80	180	2	4	6
Fish Sticks	4 sticks	200	400	18	9	10
Salted Rice Cakes	1 cake	35	75	7.3	0.7	0.3
Canned Baked Beans	1 cup	239	856	53.7	12.1	0.9
Instant Oatmeal (flavored)	1 packet	155	250	27	4	2
Feta Cheese	1 oz (28g)	75	316	1.2	4	6
Kimchi	1 cup	23	747	4	2	0.3
Sauerkraut	1 cup	27	939	6.2	1.3	0.2
Salted Tofu	1 oz (28g)	70	60	2	8	4
Miso Soup	1 cup	84	998	7	6	3
Blue Cheese	1 oz (28g)	100	395	0.7	6.1	8.1
Salted Edamame	1 cup	189	9.3	13.8	16.9	8

Canned Tuna in Brine	1 can (165g)	191	383	0	42.1	1.3
Salted Cod	3 oz (85g)	70	1900	0	15	0.5
Salted Crackers	5 crackers	80	200	10	1	3
Cheddar Cheese	1 oz (28g)	113	174	0.4	7	9.4
Salted Caramel Snacks	1 oz (28g)	135	150	20	2	5
BBQ Sauce (for dipping)	2 tbsp	60	280	14	0	0
Salted Granola Bars	1 bar	200	200	30	5	7
Canned Sardines in Oil	1 can	191	465	0	22.7	10.5
Salted Pecans	1 oz (28g)	201	0	4	2.6	20.4
Beef Tacos (fast food)	1 taco	210	500	22	10	10
Salted Walnuts	1 oz (28g)	185	1	3.9	4.3	18.5

PRINCIPLES OF ENDOMORPH DIET PLANNING

Establishing a Caloric Deficit

Embarking on a journey toward better health and fitness often leads us to confront the concept of a caloric deficit. Particularly for individuals with an endomorphic body type, understanding and effectively establishing a caloric deficit is paramount. This foundational principle is not merely about reducing calorie intake; it's about crafting a balanced approach to nutrition that supports sustainable weight loss, preserves muscle mass, and enhances overall well-being.

The Essence of a Caloric Deficit

At its core, a caloric deficit occurs when you consume fewer calories than your body expends for energy. This energy imbalance signals your body to tap into stored fat for fuel, leading to weight loss. However, the art and science of creating a caloric deficit extend beyond simple arithmetic. It involves a nuanced understanding of your body's metabolic needs, the quality of calories consumed, and how different types of foods can influence your energy levels and satiety.

Calculating Your Caloric Needs

The first step in establishing a caloric deficit is to determine your Total Daily Energy Expenditure (TDEE). This figure represents the total number of calories you burn in a day, combining your Basal Metabolic Rate (BMR)—the calories your body needs to perform basic life-sustaining functions—with the energy expended through physical activity and the thermic effect of food (TEF), which is the energy used for digestion.

Several online calculators can help you estimate your TDEE, but for a more personalized approach, consider consulting with a healthcare professional or a registered dietitian. Remember, these calculations provide a starting point. Monitoring your weight and energy levels and adjusting your caloric intake accordingly is crucial for accuracy over time.

Setting a Sustainable Caloric Deficit

A sustainable caloric deficit is one that leads to steady, manageable weight loss without compromising your health or energy levels. A common recommendation is to aim for a deficit of 500 to 750 calories per day, which typically results in a weight loss of about 1 to 1.5 pounds per week. This rate is considered safe and sustainable, reducing the risk of muscle loss and metabolic slowdown.

However, the exact deficit that works for you may vary. Factors such as your starting weight, fitness level, and daily activity must be considered. The goal is to find a balance where you're losing weight at a healthy pace while still feeling energized and satisfied.

Quality of Calories Matters

While the quantity of calories consumed is crucial for weight loss, the quality of those calories is equally important. Not all calories are created equal; 100 calories from a sugary snack can have a very different effect on your body than 100 calories from a piece of lean protein or a serving of vegetables.

Foods that are nutrient-dense and high in fiber, protein, and healthy fats tend to be more satiating and can help control hunger, making it easier to maintain a caloric deficit. They also support metabolic health, muscle maintenance, and overall well-being. In contrast, foods high in added sugars and refined carbs can spike blood sugar levels, leading to increased hunger and cravings.

Incorporating Nutrient Timing

While the focus is often on what and how much to eat, when you eat can also play a role in establishing and maintaining a caloric deficit. Nutrient timing, such as consuming protein-rich foods after a workout, can help support muscle repair and growth. Similarly, spacing your meals and snacks to manage hunger and energy levels throughout the day can prevent overeating and help sustain your caloric deficit.

The Role of Physical Activity

Physical activity is a vital component of any weight management strategy. Not only does it increase the number of calories you burn, but it also supports muscle strength, cardiovascular health, and mental well-being. For endomorphs, combining resistance training with aerobic exercises can be particularly effective. Resistance training helps build and preserve muscle mass, crucial for maintaining a healthy metabolism, while aerobic exercises increase calorie burn and improve heart health.

Adjusting and Refining Your Approach

Establishing a caloric deficit is not a "set it and forget it" strategy. It requires ongoing adjustment and refinement based on your progress, how you feel, and changes in your lifestyle or activity levels. Regularly tracking your intake, weight, and energy levels can provide valuable insights, allowing you to tweak your caloric intake and expenditure to continue making progress toward your goals.

Moreover, it's essential to listen to your body and adjust your approach if you're feeling consistently fatigued, hungry, or if your weight loss stalls. These signals can indicate that your caloric deficit is too aggressive or that you need to reassess your macronutrient balance and meal timing.

Embracing Flexibility and Compassion

Finally, while establishing a caloric deficit is critical for weight loss, it's equally important to approach this process with flexibility and self-compassion. There will be days when you exceed your calorie goal or when life circumstances make it challenging to stick to your plan. Rather than viewing these instances as failures, see them as opportunities to learn and grow. Adjusting your approach, finding what works best for you, and maintaining a positive, resilient mindset are key to long-term success.

The Importance of a Meal Plan

Embarking on a journey towards better health, weight management, or athletic performance often begins with what we choose to put on our plates. The significance of a well-structured meal plan cannot be overstated, acting as a roadmap to navigate the complex landscape of nutrition and dietetics. This discourse aims to unravel the layers of meal planning, highlighting its pivotal role in achieving and maintaining optimal health outcomes.

A Blueprint for Nutritional Success

At its core, a meal plan serves as a blueprint for nutritional success. It's a deliberate approach, meticulously designed to ensure that every meal contributes towards the overarching goals of health, fitness, and well-being. For individuals striving to manage their weight, especially those with an endomorphic body type characterized by a propensity to store fat, a meal plan is not just beneficial—it's essential.

The process of meal planning transcends the mere selection of foods; it involves a deep understanding of one's nutritional needs, preferences, and lifestyle. It's about creating a balance—ensuring that each meal is a harmonious blend of macronutrients (proteins, fats, and carbohydrates) and micronutrients (vitamins and minerals) that the body requires for optimal functioning.

Tailored to Individual Needs

One of the most compelling arguments for the adoption of a meal plan is its ability to be tailored to individual needs. No two individuals are the same; we vary in our metabolic rates, physical activity levels, and nutritional requirements. A well-crafted meal plan takes these variables into account, offering a personalized dietary strategy that aligns with one's specific health goals, whether it's weight loss, muscle gain, or improving metabolic health.

For endomorphs, who may find it challenging to lose weight due to their slower metabolism, a meal plan can be a game-changer. It can help regulate caloric intake, ensuring that calories consumed are balanced with calories expended through physical activity. Moreover, by prioritizing low-glycemic carbohydrates, lean proteins, and healthy fats, the meal plan can aid in stabilizing blood sugar levels and enhancing satiety, reducing the likelihood of overeating.

Facilitates Nutrient Timing and Portion Control

Another facet of meal planning is its role in facilitating nutrient timing and portion control—two critical components of dietary success. Nutrient timing involves consuming specific nutrients at strategic times to optimize health and performance outcomes. For instance, consuming a protein-rich meal post-exercise can enhance muscle recovery and growth. A meal plan meticulously outlines when and what to eat, taking the guesswork out of meal times and ensuring that the body receives the right nutrients at the right time.

Portion control is equally vital, particularly in a world where food portions have steadily increased. A meal plan provides a clear framework for the quantity of food to be consumed, helping to avoid the common pitfall of overeating. This is especially beneficial for endomorphs, for whom managing portion sizes can be crucial in achieving a caloric deficit for weight loss.

Promotes Dietary Diversity and Culinary Creativity

Contrary to the misconception that meal planning is restrictive, it actually promotes dietary diversity and culinary creativity. By planning meals in advance, individuals are encouraged to explore a variety of foods and recipes, ensuring a wide range of nutrients are consumed. This not only prevents nutritional deficiencies but also keeps the diet interesting and enjoyable, increasing adherence in the long term.

Moreover, meal planning can be a creative endeavor, challenging individuals to experiment with new ingredients, cooking methods, and cuisines. This exploration can lead to the discovery of new favorite dishes, expanding one's culinary repertoire and enhancing the overall dining experience.

Streamlines Grocery Shopping and Reduces Food Waste

From a practical standpoint, meal planning streamlines the grocery shopping process. With a clear list of required ingredients, individuals can shop more efficiently, avoiding impulse purchases that do not align with their dietary goals. This not only saves time but also reduces food waste, as every purchased item has a purpose within the meal plan.

Additionally, meal planning can lead to significant cost savings. By buying only what is needed and utilizing ingredients across multiple meals, individuals can minimize waste and avoid the financial drain associated with frequent takeout meals or unplanned grocery trips.

Fosters Discipline and Accountability

Lastly, the act of meal planning fosters discipline and accountability. It requires setting aside time each week to plan meals, shop for ingredients, and prepare food. This disciplined approach can spill over into other areas of life, promoting a sense of responsibility and self-accountability.

Moreover, by sticking to a meal plan, individuals are more likely to remain committed to their health and fitness goals. It serves as a constant reminder of their objectives, encouraging them to make choices that align with their desired outcomes.

Strategic Meal Timing and Frequency

In the quest for optimal health and weight management, especially for those with an endomorphic body type, understanding the nuances of meal timing and frequency can be a game-changer. This isn't just about what you eat; it's also about when and how often you eat. The strategic organization of your meals can significantly impact your metabolism, energy levels, and overall satiety, turning the tide in your favor in the battle against unwanted weight gain.

The Science of Meal Timing

The concept of meal timing revolves around synchronizing your food intake with your body's natural rhythms—known as circadian rhythms. These rhythms influence your metabolism, dictating not only how you burn calories but also how your body processes macronutrients throughout the day. For instance, research suggests that our bodies may be more efficient at processing carbohydrates earlier in the day, when our metabolic rate is higher. Conversely, late-night eating has been linked to increased body fat, as our metabolism slows down, preparing for rest.

For endomorphs, leveraging this knowledge means planning the majority of carbohydrate intake during the first half of the day, when the body is primed for higher metabolic activity. Breakfast, often touted as the most important meal of the day, should not be skipped. It kickstarts your metabolism after a night of fasting, setting a positive pace for energy use throughout the day. Including proteins and healthy fats in your morning meal can also enhance satiety, reducing the likelihood of overeating later.

The Role of Meal Frequency

The debate between eating three square meals versus several smaller meals throughout the day continues to be a topic of discussion among nutrition experts. However, the consensus leans towards a more personalized approach—what works best for your body and lifestyle.

For endomorphs, the goal is to maintain stable blood sugar levels and avoid the peaks and troughs that can lead to cravings and overeating. Eating smaller, more frequent meals can be beneficial in this regard, as it helps keep hunger at bay and provides consistent energy. This approach can also prevent the metabolic slowdown associated with large, infrequent meals, supporting a more active metabolism throughout the day.

However, it's crucial to note that "more frequent" does not mean "more food." The key is to distribute your daily caloric intake evenly across these meals, focusing on nutrient-dense foods that support your body's needs without exceeding your caloric budget.

Pre- and Post-Workout Nutrition

For individuals engaging in regular exercise—a critical component of managing an endomorphic physique—meal timing takes on an additional layer of importance. Nutrient timing, specifically around your workouts, can significantly influence your performance and recovery.

Pre-workout Nutrition: The aim here is to fuel your body for the activity ahead. A meal or snack rich in low to moderate-glycemic index carbohydrates 1-2 hours before exercise can provide a sustained energy release. Adding a moderate amount of protein can aid in muscle support without diverting too much blood to the digestive system during your workout.

Post-workout Nutrition: After exercise, your body is in a state of repair and recovery. This is the optimal time to replenish glycogen stores with carbohydrates and provide protein to aid in muscle repair. A post-workout meal or snack should be consumed within 45 minutes to an hour after exercise to maximize recovery nutrients' absorption.

Listening to Your Body

While the principles of strategic meal timing and frequency provide a framework, they are not one-size-fits-all. Individual responses can vary based on numerous factors, including age, sex, activity level, and personal health goals. Therefore, it's essential to listen to your body and adjust based on how you feel and your progress towards your goals.

For some, eating every few hours may feel natural and beneficial. For others, three well-balanced meals might be more satisfying and manageable. The key is to remain flexible and willing to adjust your approach as you learn what makes you feel your best.

Implementing the Strategy

Adopting a strategic approach to meal timing and frequency requires planning and mindfulness. Start by outlining your typical day, noting the times you naturally feel hungry and when you're most active. Use this as a blueprint to structure your meals and snacks, ensuring you're fueling your body when it needs it most.

Remember, consistency is crucial. Try to eat at similar times each day to help regulate your body's internal clock, improving metabolic efficiency over time. However, life is unpredictable, and flexibility is essential. Don't stress over occasional deviations from your plan; what matters most is the overall pattern of your eating habits.

Adjusting and Personalizing the Diet Plan

Personalization is the cornerstone of an effective diet plan. It acknowledges that we are not just a collection of metabolic processes, but individuals with tastes, preferences, and lifestyles that significantly impact our dietary choices. For endomorphs, who often face a tougher battle with weight management, personalization is not just beneficial; it's essential.

Start by assessing your dietary preferences. Do you lean towards certain cuisines or have specific dietary restrictions? Incorporating foods you enjoy and avoiding those you dislike will make your diet more enjoyable and sustainable. Remember, the goal is to create a plan that you can stick with long-term, not just for a few weeks or months.

Next, consider your lifestyle. Are you someone with a hectic schedule, or do you have more flexibility? Your diet plan should complement your daily routine, not complicate it. For busy individuals, meal prepping or choosing simple, quick recipes might be the way to go. On the other hand, if you enjoy cooking and have more time, exploring diverse and complex recipes can add excitement to your meals.

The Science of Adjustment

Adjustment is the process of fine-tuning your diet based on the feedback your body provides. It's a dynamic process that requires attention to detail and a willingness to experiment. Start by monitoring your progress. This can be done through various means such as tracking your weight, taking body measurements, or noting changes in how your clothes fit.

Pay attention to how you feel as well. Increased energy levels, improved sleep quality, and a general sense of well-being are all positive signs that your diet is working for you. Conversely, feelings of lethargy, irritability, or persistent hunger may indicate that adjustments are needed.

One common adjustment is caloric intake. If you're not seeing the desired weight loss, you may need to create a larger caloric deficit either by reducing your intake or increasing your physical activity. Conversely, if you're losing weight too quickly or feeling constantly fatigued, it might be time to increase your calories to support your body's needs.

Macronutrient ratios are another area ripe for adjustment. While a lower carbohydrate, higher protein diet may work well for many endomorphs, it's not a one-size-fits-all solution. Some may find they perform better with a slightly higher carbohydrate intake, especially if they're very active. Listen to your body and adjust accordingly.

Overcoming Plateaus and Setbacks

Plateaus are a common and frustrating part of any weight loss journey. They occur when, despite following your diet and exercise plan, your weight loss stalls. First, assess whether you're truly at a plateau or if normal weight fluctuations are masking progress. If it's a plateau, consider mixing up your routine. This could mean changing your workout regimen, adjusting your caloric intake, or altering your macronutrient ratios.

Setbacks, on the other hand, are inevitable. Life happens, and there will be times when you stray from your diet plan. The key is not to view these moments as failures but as opportunities to learn and grow. Reflect on what led to the setback and how you can better prepare for similar situations in the future. Remember, consistency over perfection is what leads to long-term success.

Embracing Flexibility

A personalized diet plan is not set in stone; it's a living document that evolves as you do. Embrace flexibility in your approach. Celebrate your successes, learn from your setbacks, and always be willing to make the necessary adjustments. This flexibility not only applies to what you eat but how you eat. Some days you might find yourself hungrier than usual, or you may have social events that don't fit neatly into your plan. Learning to navigate these situations without guilt or stress is crucial for long-term success.

Meal Planning and Preparation Tips for Endomorphs

Embarking on a journey to manage weight and improve overall health can be a transformative experience, especially for individuals with an endomorphic body type. Endomorphs, characterized by a propensity to store fat, a slower metabolism, and a sturdy build, often face unique challenges in achieving their fitness goals. However, with the right meal planning and preparation strategies, overcoming these hurdles becomes not just possible, but enjoyable. This guide aims to arm you with practical, effective tips for meal planning and preparation that cater specifically to the needs of endomorphs, ensuring your path to wellness is both successful and sustainable.

Understanding the Endomorph Diet

Before diving into meal planning and preparation, it's crucial to understand the dietary needs unique to endomorphs. A diet that balances macronutrients—lower in carbohydrates, higher in protein, and moderate in fats—can help manage weight and support metabolic health. Emphasizing whole, nutrient-dense foods while minimizing processed foods and sugars is key. With this foundation, let's explore how to translate these principles into a practical meal plan.

Setting Clear Goals

Begin by setting clear, achievable goals. Whether it's losing weight, gaining muscle, or simply improving overall health, your goals will guide your meal planning process. Be specific about what you want to achieve and by when, as this will help you stay focused and motivated.

Planning Your Meals

1. **Weekly Meal Planning**: Dedicate time each week to plan your meals. This includes breakfast, lunch, dinner, and any snacks. Planning ahead prevents last-minute unhealthy choices and ensures you have all the necessary ingredients on hand.

2. **Macronutrient Balance**: For each meal, aim for a balance of macronutrients. Incorporate lean proteins, healthy fats, and low-glycemic carbohydrates to keep you full and energized throughout the day. For example, a meal might include grilled chicken (protein), a side of quinoa (carbohydrates), and avocado (fat).

3. **Portion Control**: Understanding portion sizes is crucial. Use measuring cups, a food scale, or visual cues (e.g., a fist-sized portion of carbs) to ensure you're eating the right amounts for your goals.

4. **Diverse Menu**: Variety is the spice of life and a key to nutritional success. Rotate your protein sources, vegetables, and whole grains to prevent boredom and ensure you're getting a range of nutrients.

Preparation Tips

1. **Batch Cooking**: Prepare meals in bulk to save time and ensure you have healthy options readily available. Cook a large batch of protein, like chicken or tofu, and a whole grain, like brown rice or quinoa, at the beginning of the week.

2. **Smart Snacking**: Prepare healthy snacks in advance to avoid reaching for convenient, less nutritious options. Cut vegetables and portion out hummus, prepare fruit and yogurt parfaits, or make a batch of protein balls.

3. **Invest in Quality Containers**: Good-quality, portion-controlled containers are invaluable. They make it easy to store and transport meals, keeping them fresh and appetizing.

4. **Spice It Up**: Keep a variety of spices and herbs on hand to add flavor without extra calories. Experimenting with different seasonings can make even the simplest meals exciting.

5. **Hydration**: Don't forget about water. Staying well-hydrated is essential for metabolism and overall health. Keep a water bottle with you at all times and consider infusing your water with fruits or herbs for variety.

Overcoming Challenges

Meal planning and preparation can seem daunting at first, especially for busy individuals. However, by incorporating these strategies into your routine, you'll find it becomes second nature:

- **Time Management**: Set aside specific times for meal planning, shopping, and preparation. Treat these as non-negotiable appointments with yourself.

- **Simplify Where Needed**: Not every meal needs to be a culinary masterpiece. Simple, nutritious meals are often the most satisfying and easiest to prepare.

- **Involve Family or Roommates**: Make meal planning and preparation a shared activity. It's more enjoyable and can help you stay committed to your goals.

- **Adapt and Adjust**: Be prepared to adjust your meal plan based on your progress, feedback from your body, and changes in your schedule or appetite.

METABOLIC CONFUSION STRATEGIES

Cyclical Caloric Rotation

The concept of cyclical caloric rotation emerges as a sophisticated strategy designed to outsmart the body's natural tendency to adapt to consistent dietary patterns. This method, part of the broader metabolic confusion approach, involves alternating between periods of higher and lower calorie intake. The goal is to prevent metabolic slowdown, a common adversary in long-term weight management efforts, and to potentially enhance fat loss while preserving lean muscle mass. Let's delve into the intricacies of cyclical caloric rotation, exploring its mechanisms, benefits, and how to implement it effectively.

Understanding the Mechanism

The human body is remarkably adept at adapting to its environment, including dietary intake. When calories are consistently restricted, the body can adjust its metabolic rate downward to conserve energy, a survival mechanism honed through millennia. Cyclical caloric rotation aims to circumvent this adaptation by varying calorie intake in a planned manner, thus keeping the metabolism active and engaged. By oscillating between higher and lower calorie days, the body is continually prompted to adjust, potentially maintaining a higher metabolic rate over time.

The Benefits of Cyclical Caloric Rotation

1. **Prevents Metabolic Stagnation**: Regularly changing calorie intake helps avoid the metabolic plateau often encountered in traditional dieting, where weight loss stalls as the body becomes more efficient at utilizing fewer calories.

2. **Enhances Fat Loss While Preserving Muscle**: Higher calorie days help support muscle maintenance and growth by ensuring adequate energy and nutrient intake, crucial for muscle repair and synthesis. Lower calorie days promote fat loss by creating a calorie deficit.

3. **Improves Dietary Adherence**: The flexibility of having higher calorie days can improve overall satisfaction and adherence to the diet, reducing the psychological strain associated with continuous calorie restriction.

4. **Supports Hormonal Balance**: Strategic higher calorie intake, especially with an emphasis on carbohydrates, can positively influence hormones like leptin and ghrelin, which regulate hunger and satiety, and cortisol, which is associated with stress and fat storage.

Implementing Cyclical Caloric Rotation

To effectively implement this strategy, a thoughtful and personalized approach is required. Here's how to get started:

1. **Determine Your Caloric Needs**: First, calculate your Total Daily Energy Expenditure (TDEE), which is the number of calories you need to maintain your current weight. Numerous online calculators can help you estimate this figure based on your age, gender, weight, height, and activity level.

2. **Set Your Caloric Range**: Decide on your lower and higher calorie targets. On lower calorie days, aim for a reduction of 20-30% below your TDEE to promote fat loss. On higher calorie days, you can go up to maintenance level or slightly above to support metabolic activity and muscle recovery.

3. **Plan Your Rotation Schedule**: The frequency and pattern of rotation can vary based on personal preference, goals, and lifestyle. A common approach is to align higher calorie days with more intense training days, providing the body with more fuel for exercise and recovery. A simple pattern might involve three lower calorie days followed by one higher calorie day, but this can be adjusted as needed.

4. **Focus on Nutrient Quality**: Regardless of high or low calorie days, the quality of your calories matters. Prioritize whole, nutrient-dense foods that provide ample protein, healthy fats, and complex carbohydrates. Even on higher calorie days, avoid the temptation to fill up on empty calories from highly processed foods.

5. **Monitor and Adjust**: Regularly assess your progress and how your body is responding. Adjustments may be necessary based on changes in weight, energy levels, and overall well-being. Flexibility is a key component of cyclical caloric rotation, allowing for modifications to better suit your evolving needs.

Practical Tips for Success

- **Stay Hydrated**: Proper hydration is crucial for metabolic health and can help manage hunger on lower calorie days.

- **Incorporate Variety**: Keep your diet interesting by experimenting with different foods and recipes that meet your nutritional goals, reducing the risk of dietary boredom.

- **Listen to Your Body**: Pay attention to how your body responds to different caloric levels, adjusting as necessary to optimize energy, performance, and satisfaction.

Macronutrient Shifting

The concept of macronutrient shifting emerges as a sophisticated strategy designed to optimize body composition, enhance metabolic efficiency, and break through weight loss plateaus. This approach, rooted in the principle of metabolic flexibility, involves varying the ratios of carbohydrates, proteins, and fats in your diet over different periods. The goal is to leverage the unique metabolic pathways activated by each macronutrient to fuel performance, recovery, and fat loss. Let's delve into the intricacies of macronutrient shifting and how you can implement this strategy effectively.

Understanding Macronutrients

Before we explore the dynamics of macronutrient shifting, a brief overview of the roles of carbohydrates, proteins, and fats is essential. Carbohydrates are the body's primary energy source, particularly for high-intensity activities. Proteins are crucial for muscle repair, growth, and various bodily functions. Fats, dense in calories, support hormone production, cellular health, and provide a sustained energy source. Each macronutrient plays a pivotal role in our health, and altering their intake can significantly impact our body's functioning.

The Rationale behind Macronutrient Shifting

The underlying premise of macronutrient shifting is to prevent the body from adapting to a static nutritional environment. By periodically adjusting macronutrient ratios, you can stimulate different metabolic processes, potentially enhancing fat oxidation, improving insulin sensitivity, and supporting lean muscle mass. This strategy not only aids in weight management but also aligns with the body's varying nutritional needs based on activity levels, goals, and physiological responses.

Implementing Macronutrient Shifting

1. **Identify Your Goals**: Whether you aim to lose fat, build muscle, or improve athletic performance, your objectives will dictate how you adjust your macronutrient ratios. For instance, increasing protein and reducing carbohydrates may be beneficial for fat loss, while boosting carbohydrates is advantageous for endurance athletes.

2. **Understand Your Baseline**: Establish your daily caloric needs and current macronutrient distribution. This baseline serves as your starting point for implementing shifts.

3. **Plan Your Shifts**: Decide on the pattern of your macronutrient shifts. Some individuals prefer weekly cycles, adjusting their intake based on the intensity of their training schedule, while others may opt for longer phases, such as a month focused on building muscle followed by a period of fat loss.

4. **Monitor and Adjust**: Pay close attention to how your body responds to these shifts. Use indicators such as body composition, energy levels, workout performance, and overall well-being to gauge effectiveness. Be prepared to adjust your approach based on these feedback mechanisms.

Strategies for Macronutrient Shifting

- **Carb Cycling**: This popular method involves alternating between high-carb days (usually on heavy training days) and low-carb days (on rest or light activity days). The aim is to fuel intense workouts and recovery while promoting fat loss on low-carb days.
- **Protein Pulsing**: Increase your protein intake on days you engage in strength training to support muscle repair and growth. On rest days, you can slightly reduce protein intake, though it should still remain a significant part of your diet.
- **Fat Focused**: On days when carbohydrate intake is lower, increase your healthy fat intake to maintain energy levels and support hormone health. This approach is particularly useful during lower-intensity training phases or rest days.

Benefits of Macronutrient Shifting

- **Enhanced Metabolic Flexibility**: By regularly altering your macronutrient intake, you can improve your body's ability to switch between using carbohydrates and fats as fuel, enhancing energy efficiency and fat loss.
- **Prevents Dietary Monotony**: Changing your macronutrient ratios keeps your diet interesting, increasing the likelihood of adherence over the long term.
- **Aligned with Physiological Needs**: Macronutrient shifting allows for nutritional intake to be more closely aligned with the body's fluctuating needs, supporting optimal performance and recovery.

Intermittent Fasting Variations

Intermittent fasting (IF) has surged in popularity as a flexible approach to eating that can complement various lifestyles and health goals. Unlike traditional diets that focus on *what* to eat, intermittent fasting concentrates on *when* to eat, providing a framework that can lead to improved metabolic health, weight loss, and even enhanced longevity. This guide explores the variations of intermittent fasting, offering insights into how each method can be tailored to fit individual needs and preferences.

Understanding Intermittent Fasting

At its core, intermittent fasting involves cycling between periods of eating and fasting. This practice isn't new; it echoes the eating patterns of our ancestors, who didn't have access to food around the clock. Modern research suggests that these periods of fasting can trigger numerous beneficial processes in the body, such as improved insulin sensitivity, increased growth hormone levels, and enhanced cellular repair mechanisms.

The Variations of Intermittent Fasting

Each variation of intermittent fasting offers unique benefits and challenges, making it crucial to select the method that aligns with your lifestyle, health status, and goals. Here are the most popular IF protocols:

1. **The 16/8 Method**: Also known as the Leangains protocol, this method involves fasting for 16 hours each day and eating all your meals within an 8-hour window. For many, this means skipping breakfast and eating from noon to 8 p.m. This approach is particularly favored for its simplicity and ease of integration into daily life.

2. **The 5:2 Diet**: This approach requires eating normally for five days of the week while restricting calories to 500-600 on the other two days, which are not consecutive. The 5:2 diet appeals to those who prefer not to fast completely but are capable of significant calorie reduction on specific days.

3. **Eat-Stop-Eat**: Involves a 24-hour fast once or twice a week. For example, not eating from dinner one day until dinner the next day. This method can be more challenging due to the longer fasting periods but is effective for those seeking to reduce calorie intake significantly.

4. **The Warrior Diet**: This diet mimics the eating patterns of ancient warriors, consisting of small amounts of raw fruits and vegetables during the day and one large meal at night. The Warrior Diet is designed for those interested in combining aspects of fasting with a focus on whole, unprocessed foods.

5. **Alternate-Day Fasting (ADF)**: As the name suggests, this involves alternating between days of normal eating and days of either complete fasting or consuming a minimal amount of calories (about 500). ADF can be quite effective but may require a higher level of discipline and adjustment.

6. **The 12-Hour Fast**: A gentler approach, this method simply extends the natural overnight fasting period to 12 hours. For many, this means finishing dinner by 7 p.m. and not eating again until 7 a.m. It's an excellent starting point for beginners to intermittent fasting.

Tailoring Intermittent Fasting to Your Lifestyle

Choosing the right intermittent fasting method depends on your daily routine, health goals, and how your body responds to fasting. Consider the following when selecting a fasting protocol:

- **Lifestyle Compatibility**: Select a fasting method that fits seamlessly into your daily routine. For instance, if skipping breakfast works well for you, the 16/8 method might be ideal.
- **Health Goals**: Are you looking to lose weight, improve metabolic health, or enhance longevity? Different fasting methods can have varying effects, so align your choice with your objectives.
- **Personal Preferences**: Consider your ability to handle longer periods without food. If you find it challenging, starting with a shorter fasting window like the 12-hour fast may be beneficial.

Maximizing the Benefits of Intermittent Fasting

To fully reap the benefits of intermittent fasting, consider these tips:

- **Stay Hydrated**: Drink plenty of water throughout the day, especially during fasting periods, to stay hydrated and help curb hunger.
- **Nutrient-Dense Foods**: When you do eat, focus on nutrient-dense foods that provide vitamins, minerals, and antioxidants to support your overall health.
- **Listen to Your Body**: Pay attention to how your body responds to fasting. If a particular method causes discomfort or stress, consider trying a different approach.
- **Combine with Healthy Lifestyle Choices**: Intermittent fasting is most effective when combined with other healthy habits, such as regular physical activity, adequate sleep, and stress management.

Periodic Refeeding Days

The concept of periodic refeeding days emerges as a strategic tool designed to counteract the metabolic slowdown associated with prolonged calorie restriction. This approach not only reinvigorates the metabolism but also addresses the psychological challenges of dieting, offering a structured reprieve from the rigors of calorie counting. Let's delve into the science, benefits, and practical implementation of periodic refeeding days, providing a comprehensive guide for those looking to optimize their weight loss journey.

The Science behind Refeeding

Periodic refeeding involves intentionally increasing calorie intake, particularly from carbohydrates, for a short duration, typically one to two days, after a period of calorie restriction. This practice is grounded in its ability to stimulate leptin, a hormone responsible for regulating hunger and energy expenditure. During periods of calorie restriction, leptin levels drop, signaling the body to conserve energy and potentially slowing down metabolism. A refeed boosts leptin levels, temporarily enhancing metabolic rate and creating a more favorable environment for fat loss.

The Dual Benefits of Refeeding

Metabolic Revitalization: By strategically increasing calorie intake, refeeding days can help mitigate the metabolic adaptation that often accompanies weight loss. This adaptation, while evolutionarily beneficial, can be a hindrance to modern-day weight loss efforts, making it increasingly difficult to lose weight over time. Refeeding days help "reset" the metabolism, keeping it more active and responsive.

Psychological Relief: Dieting, especially for extended periods, can be mentally taxing. The restrictive nature of calorie counting can lead to feelings of deprivation, which can undermine motivation and adherence. Refeeding days offer a psychological break, allowing individuals to enjoy a wider variety of foods and temporarily relax dietary restrictions. This can improve overall diet satisfaction and sustainability.

Implementing Refeeding Days

Timing and Frequency: The optimal timing and frequency of refeeding days depend on several factors, including the individual's metabolic rate, the extent of calorie restriction, and physical activity levels. Generally, a refeed every 1-2 weeks is a good starting point for those on a moderate calorie deficit. Those on a more aggressive diet or with higher levels of physical activity may benefit from more frequent refeeds.

Caloric and Macronutrient Considerations: On a refeed day, the goal is to increase caloric intake by 20-30% above maintenance levels, with a focus on carbohydrates. Carbohydrates are particularly effective at raising leptin levels. It's important to source these additional calories from high-quality, nutrient-dense carbohydrates like whole grains, fruits, and vegetables, rather than sugary foods or refined carbs.

Continued Protein and Fat Intake: While the emphasis is on carbohydrates, maintaining adequate protein intake is crucial for muscle preservation, especially in a calorie-restricted regimen. Fats should still be included but can be slightly reduced to accommodate the increase in carbohydrates.

Monitoring and Adjusting: As with any dietary strategy, the key to success with refeeding days is monitoring and adjustment. Pay attention to how your body responds in terms of hunger, energy levels, and weight loss progress. Adjust the frequency and magnitude of refeeds based on these observations and your overall goals.

Maximizing the Benefits of Refeeding Days

Plan Ahead: To make the most of refeeding days, plan them in advance. This allows you to ensure that you have the right foods available and can align refeeds with social events or workouts, maximizing enjoyment and utility.

Stay Mindful: While refeeding days are a break from strict calorie counting, they're not an excuse for unbridled overeating. Focus on enjoying your meals mindfully, savoring the flavors, and listening to your body's hunger and fullness cues.

Incorporate Resistance Training: Aligning refeeding days with heavy resistance training sessions can enhance muscle glycogen replenishment and support muscle synthesis, leveraging the increased calorie intake for muscle growth and repair.

Evaluate Progress Holistically: When incorporating refeeding days into your diet plan, assess your progress holistically. Look beyond the scale, considering changes in body composition, energy levels, workout performance, and overall well-being.

Weekly Caloric Distribution Adjustment

This approach, rooted in the principles of metabolic flexibility, offers a dynamic pathway to achieving weight loss goals while catering to the body's varying energy demands. By understanding and implementing this strategy, individuals can navigate their dietary journey with greater ease and effectiveness.

The Foundation of Weekly Caloric Distribution

Weekly caloric distribution adjustment is predicated on the understanding that our bodies' energy needs fluctuate daily based on activity levels, hormonal changes, and metabolic demands. Traditional diet plans often overlook this variability, prescribing a static calorie intake that may not align with the body's actual requirements. In contrast, weekly caloric distribution adjustment allows for a more nuanced approach, allocating calories in a way that supports metabolic health, encourages fat loss, and preserves muscle mass.

Strategic Implementation

1. **Understanding Your Caloric Baseline**: The first step involves calculating your total daily energy expenditure (TDEE), which is the sum of your basal metabolic rate (BMR), the thermic effect of food (TEF), and energy expended through physical activity. This figure represents your maintenance calories—the amount needed to maintain your current weight.

2. **Setting a Weekly Goal**: Once your TDEE is established, determine your weekly caloric deficit goal based on your weight loss objectives. A reasonable starting point is a deficit of 3,500 to 7,000 calories per week, translating to 1-2 pounds of weight loss, as this range is generally considered safe and sustainable.

3. **Distributing Calories Across the Week**: With your weekly goal in mind, distribute your calories in a way that aligns with your lifestyle and activity levels. For instance, allocate more calories on days you engage in strenuous physical activities and fewer on sedentary days. This not only fuels your workouts effectively but also aids in recovery and muscle synthesis.

4. **Incorporating Flexibility**: The beauty of this approach lies in its flexibility. Life is unpredictable, and social events, work commitments, or changes in workout intensity can all impact your daily calorie needs. Weekly caloric distribution adjustment allows you to "borrow" calories from one day to compensate for another, ensuring you stay on track without sacrificing your social life or well-being.

Advantages of Weekly Caloric Distribution Adjustment

- **Enhanced Metabolic Flexibility**: By varying your calorie intake, you may improve your body's ability to switch between fuel sources efficiently, potentially boosting metabolism and enhancing fat loss.

- **Psychological Benefits**: This method introduces dietary flexibility, reducing the mental strain associated with strict daily calorie limits. It accommodates life's ebb and flow, making your diet plan more sustainable and enjoyable.

- **Improved Nutritional Outcomes**: Allocating more calories to active days ensures you're adequately fueled for your workouts, supporting better performance and recovery. On rest days, reducing calorie intake can aid in fat loss without compromising muscle mass.

Practical Tips for Success

- **Plan Ahead**: Spend time each week planning your meals and snacks. This foresight ensures you can adjust your caloric intake based on your anticipated activity levels and commitments.

- **Track Your Intake**: Utilize a food diary or an app to monitor your daily and weekly calorie consumption. This data is invaluable for making informed adjustments to your diet plan.

- **Listen to Your Body**: Pay attention to hunger cues and energy levels. If you find yourself consistently hungry or fatigued, you may need to reassess your caloric distribution or overall deficit.

- **Stay Hydrated**: Proper hydration is crucial for metabolic health and appetite regulation. Ensure you're drinking enough water, especially on higher calorie, more active days.

- **Seek Nutrient Density**: Focus on filling your plate with nutrient-dense foods—vegetables, fruits, lean proteins, whole grains, and healthy fats. These foods provide the vitamins, minerals, and fiber your body needs to thrive, especially when operating on a calorie deficit.

CONCLUSION

Embarking on the journey of better health and fitness, especially for those with an endomorphic body type, can often feel like navigating through a labyrinth of conflicting advice and fleeting trends. The "Metabolic Confusion Diet Food List for Endomorphs" stands as a beacon of hope, promising not just a transformation in how we engage with food and understand our metabolism but also offering a tailored path toward optimal health for endomorphs. This meticulously curated guide is more than a compilation of foods; it's a compass that guides through the principles of metabolic confusion, specifically tailored for the endomorph body type.

The essence of metabolic confusion lies in its strategic approach to dieting, which deviates from the monotonous calorie-counting and restrictive eating habits that have long dominated the dieting landscape. By embracing the uniqueness of each individual's metabolic blueprint, the diet acknowledges that the endomorph body type has specific needs and responses to food. This realization is empowering, marking the beginning of a personalized nutrition journey that speaks directly to your body's unique language.

The book delves into the scientific underpinnings that make metabolic confusion a viable strategy for overcoming weight loss plateaus, enhancing metabolic flexibility, and fostering a healthier relationship with food. By alternating between periods of higher and lower calorie intake, the metabolism is encouraged to remain in a state of gentle flux, optimizing fat loss and muscle gain without the stagnation often encountered in traditional diets.

Moreover, the journey toward health is recognized as much about the mental and emotional aspects as it is about the physical. The frustration stemming from following diet after diet, only to find oneself back at square one, is a cycle many have endured. This book aims to break that cycle by introducing variety, flexibility, and personalization into your diet, rekindling your enthusiasm for nourishment and making eating a joyous and life-affirming act rather than a source of stress.

Within these pages, you will find not just a list of foods but a comprehensive exploration of macronutrient balance, nutrient timing, and portion control, offering practical strategies that can be seamlessly integrated into your daily life. The goal is to foster a sense of empowerment, enabling you to make informed decisions about your diet that align with your body type, lifestyle, and personal preferences.

As you embark on this journey with the "Metabolic Confusion Diet Food List for Endomorphs," remember that this book is designed to be a living document, one that you can return to time and again, finding new insights and inspirations as you progress along your path to wellness. It's a testament to the belief that with the right knowledge and tools, anyone can unlock their body's potential for vibrant health.

We approach the topic of metabolic confusion and endomorph nutrition with a blend of scientific rigor and empathetic understanding. It's a dialogue between us, rooted in the latest research and clinical insights, yet communicated with the warmth and clarity of a trusted friend. We're here to demystify the complexities of metabolism and dieting, presenting information in a way that's accessible, relatable, and, above all, actionable.

As you turn the pages of this guide, we invite you to embark on this journey with an open mind and a committed heart. Your path to wellness is uniquely yours, and with the "Metabolic Confusion Diet Food List for Endomorphs," you have a companion tailored to illuminate the way.

Thank you for choosing to embark on this journey with us. We hope you find the insights and strategies within these pages both enlightening and empowering. Your feedback is invaluable to us, and we encourage you to leave an honest review on Amazon. Sharing your experience can not only help us improve but also inspire others to take the first step toward their health and wellness goals. Together, let's revolutionize the way we understand and engage with food, metabolism, and our bodies.

INTERACTIVE WORKSHEETS

Macronutrient Balance Tracker

Objective: To prevent metabolic adaptation and promote fat loss by varying daily caloric intake and macronutrient ratios throughout the week.

Personal Information

- **Name:** ____
- **Date:** ____
- **Starting Weight:** _______________________________________
- **Goal Weight:** ____

Weekly Caloric & Macronutrient Goals

- **High Calorie Days (HCD):** 3 days/week
  - **Calories:** _______________________________________
  - **Protein (%):** ____________________________________
  - **Carbohydrates (%):** ______________________________
  - **Fats (%):** _______________________________________
- **Low Calorie Days (LCD):** 4 days/week
  - **Calories:** _______________________________________
  - **Protein (%):** ____________________________________
  - **Carbohydrates (%):** ______________________________
  - **Fats (%):** _______________________________________

Daily Meal Planner

Day	Meal 1 (Breakfast)	Meal 2 (Snack)	Meal 3 (Lunch)	Meal 4 (Snack)	Meal 5 (Dinner)	Meal 6 (Snack)
Monday (LCD)						
Tuesday (HCD)						

Wednesday (LCD)			84			
Thursday (HCD)						
Friday (LCD)						
Saturday (HCD)						
Sunday (LCD)						

Notes & Adjustments

- **Week 1 Observations:**

  -
  -

- **Adjustments for Next Week:**

  -
  -

Weekly Caloric & Macronutrient Goals

- **High Calorie Days (HCD):** 3 days/week
    - **Calories:** _______________________________________
    - **Protein (%):** _______________________________________
    - **Carbohydrates (%):** _______________________________________
    - **Fats (%):** _______________________________________
- **Low Calorie Days (LCD):** 4 days/week
    - **Calories:** _______________________________________
    - **Protein (%):** _______________________________________
    - **Carbohydrates (%):** _______________________________________
    - **Fats (%):** _______________________________________

Daily Meal Planner

Day	Meal 1 (Breakfast)	Meal 2 (Snack)	Meal 3 (Lunch)	Meal 4 (Snack)	Meal 5 (Dinner)	Meal 6 (Snack)
Monday (LCD)						
Tuesday (HCD)						
Wednesday (LCD)						
Thursday (HCD)						
Friday (LCD)						

Saturday (HCD)			86			
Sunday (LCD)						

Notes & Adjustments

- **Week 1 Observations:**

    -
    -

- **Adjustments for Next Week:**

    -

Weekly Caloric & Macronutrient Goals

- **High Calorie Days (HCD):** 3 days/week
    - **Calories:** _______________________________________
    - **Protein (%):** _______________________________________
    - **Carbohydrates (%):** _______________________________________
    - **Fats (%):** _______________________________________
- **Low Calorie Days (LCD):** 4 days/week
    - **Calories:** _______________________________________
    - **Protein (%):** _______________________________________
    - **Carbohydrates (%):** _______________________________________
    - **Fats (%):** _______________________________________

Daily Meal Planner

Day	Meal 1 (Breakfast)	Meal 2 (Snack)	Meal 3 (Lunch)	Meal 4 (Snack)	Meal 5 (Dinner)	Meal 6 (Snack)
Monday (LCD)						
Tuesday (HCD)						
Wednesday (LCD)						
Thursday (HCD)						
Friday (LCD)						

Saturday (HCD)					
Sunday (LCD)					

Notes & Adjustments

- **Week 1 Observations:**

    -
    -

- **Adjustments for Next Week:**

    -

Weekly Caloric & Macronutrient Goals

- **High Calorie Days (HCD):** 3 days/week

  - **Calories:** ____

  - **Protein (%):** ____

  - **Carbohydrates (%):** _______________________________________

  - **Fats (%):** ____

- **Low Calorie Days (LCD):** 4 days/week

  - **Calories:** ____

  - **Protein (%):** ____

  - **Carbohydrates (%):** _______________________________________

  - **Fats (%):** ____

Daily Meal Planner

Day	Meal 1 (Breakfast)	Meal 2 (Snack)	Meal 3 (Lunch)	Meal 4 (Snack)	Meal 5 (Dinner)	Meal 6 (Snack)
Monday (LCD)						
Tuesday (HCD)						
Wednesday (LCD)						
Thursday (HCD)						
Friday (LCD)						

Saturday (HCD)			90		
Sunday (LCD)					

Notes & Adjustments

- **Week 1 Observations:**

    -

    -

- **Adjustments for Next Week:**

    -

Strength Training Log

Name: _______________________________

Date: _______________________________

Week Of: _______________________________

Goal: _______________________________

Workout Plan Overview

Day	**Muscle Group(s)**	**Exercise 1**	**Sets**	**Reps**	**Weight**	**Exercise 2**	**Sets**	**Reps**	**Weight**
Monday									
Tuesday									
Wednesday									
Thursday									
Friday									
Saturday									
Sunday									

Notes:

____

____

____

Weekly Progress Tracker

Week Ending	Total Weight Lifted	Progress Notes	Adjustments for Next Week

Personal Bests:

Reflections and Goals for Next Week:

Day	Muscle Group(s)	Exercise 1	Sets	Reps	Weight	Exercise 2	Sets	Reps	Weight
Monday									
Tuesday									
Wednesday									
Thursday									
Friday									
Saturday									
Sunday									

Notes:

____

____

____

Weekly Progress Tracker

Week Ending	Total Weight Lifted	Progress Notes	Adjustments for Next Week

Personal Bests:

____

____

Reflections and Goals for Next Week:

____

____

Workout Plan Overview

Day	Muscle Group(s)	Exercise 1	Sets	Reps	Weight	Exercise 2	Sets	Reps	Weight
Monday									
Tuesday									
Wednesday									
Thursday									
Friday									
Saturday									
Sunday									

Notes:

____

____

____

Weekly Progress Tracker

Week Ending	Total Weight Lifted	Progress Notes	Adjustments for Next Week

Personal Bests:

Reflections and Goals for Next Week:

Workout Plan Overview

Day	Muscle Group(s)	Exercise 1	Sets	Reps	Weight	Exercise 2	Sets	Reps	Weight
Monday									
Tuesday									
Wednesday									
Thursday									
Friday									
Saturday									
Sunday									

Notes:

Weekly Progress Tracker

Week Ending	Total Weight Lifted	Progress Notes	Adjustments for Next Week

Personal Bests:

Reflections and Goals for Next Week:

Cardiovascular Exercise Planner

Name: ___________________________________

Date: ______________________

Goal Setting:

- **Weekly Cardio Goal (in minutes):** ___________________
- **Types of Cardio Preferred:** _______________________
- **Intensity Level (Low, Moderate, High):** ______________

Weekly Schedule:

Day	Exercise Type (e.g., Walking, Cycling)	Duration (Minutes)	Intensity	Notes (e.g., Indoor/Outdoor, Treadmill Incline)
Monday				
Tuesday				
Wednesday				
Thursday				
Friday				
Saturday				
Sunday				

Progress Tracking:

Week Ending	Total Minutes Achieved	Notes (e.g., Adjustments, Challenges)

Reflection:

- **What worked well this week?**

- **What challenges did I face and how can I overcome them?**

- **Adjustments for Next Week:**

Signature: _______________________________

Date: _________________

Weekly Schedule:

Day	Exercise Type (e.g., Walking, Cycling)	Duration (Minutes)	Intensity	Notes (e.g., Indoor/Outdoor, Treadmill Incline)
Monday				
Tuesday				
Wednesday				
Thursday				
Friday				
Saturday				
Sunday				

Progress Tracking:

Week Ending	Total Minutes Achieved	Notes (e.g., Adjustments, Challenges)

Reflection:

- **What worked well this week?**

- **What challenges did I face and how can I overcome them?**

- **Adjustments for Next Week:**

Signature: _______________________________

Date: ___________________

Weekly Schedule:

Day	Exercise Type (e.g., Walking, Cycling)	Duration (Minutes)	Intensity	Notes (e.g., Indoor/Outdoor, Treadmill Incline)
Monday				
Tuesday				
Wednesday				
Thursday				
Friday				
Saturday				
Sunday				

Progress Tracking:

Week Ending	Total Minutes Achieved	Notes (e.g., Adjustments, Challenges)

Reflection:

- **What worked well this week?**

- **What challenges did I face and how can I overcome them?**

- **Adjustments for Next Week:**

Signature: _______________________________

Date: _______________

Weekly Schedule:

Day	Exercise Type (e.g., Walking, Cycling)	Duration (Minutes)	Intensity	Notes (e.g., Indoor/Outdoor, Treadmill Incline)
Monday				
Tuesday				
Wednesday				
Thursday				
Friday				
Saturday				
Sunday				

Progress Tracking:

Week Ending	Total Minutes Achieved	Notes (e.g., Adjustments, Challenges)

Reflection:

- **What worked well this week?**

- **What challenges did I face and how can I overcome them?**

- **Adjustments for Next Week:**

Signature: _______________________________

Date: _____________________

Stress Management and Sleep Journal

Name: ________________________

Week of: ________________________

Daily Stress Level Tracking

Date	Stress Level (1-10)	Main Stressors	Stress Reduction Techniques Used	Effectiveness (1-10)

Stress Level (1-10): 1 being the least stressed, 10 being the most stressed.

Effectiveness: 1 being not effective at all, 10 being highly effective.

Daily Sleep Journal

Date	Bedtime	Wake Time	Total Sleep Hours	Sleep Quality (1-10)	Notes (Dreams, Wake-ups)

Sleep Quality (1-10): 1 being very poor quality, 10 being excellent quality.

1. **What were the main sources of stress this week?**

____

____

____

2. **Which stress reduction techniques were most effective?**

____

____

____

2. **How did your sleep quality affect your stress levels and vice versa?**

____

____

____

3. **Goals for next week (stress reduction and sleep improvement):**

____

____

____

Hydration and Supplement Tracker

Hydration and Supplement Tracker

Name: ________________________ **Date:** ________________________

Hydration Log

Time	Amount (ml)	Notes (e.g., before/after exercise)
07:00		
09:00		
11:00		
13:00		
15:00		
17:00		
19:00		
21:00		

Daily Total: ____________ ml

Goal: Aim for at least 2-3 liters of water per day, adjusting based on activity level and personal health needs.

Supplement Log

Time	Supplement	Dosage	Purpose	Effects Noticed
07:00				
12:00				
18:00				

Note: Include vitamins, minerals, protein powders, or any other supplements you're taking.

Weekly Reflection

1. How did you feel this week in terms of hydration? Did you notice any changes in your energy levels, appetite, or physical performance?

____

____

2. How effective do you feel your current supplement regimen is? Have you noticed any improvements or side effects?

____

____

3. Any adjustments you plan to make for the next week (e.g., increasing water intake, modifying supplement types or dosages)?

____

____

My Grocery List

Day :
Month :

No.	Foods & Meals	Qty.	Notes

My Grocery List

Day :
Month :

No.	Foods & Meals	Qty.	Notes

My Grocery List

Day :

Month :

No.	Foods	Qty.	No.	Drinks	Qty.

Notes :

My Grocery List

Day :
Month :

No.	Foods	Qty.

No.	Drinks	Qty.

No.	Beverages	Qty.

No.	Snacks	Qty.

Notes :

9 798320 659893